Racing Uphill

Racing Uphill

Confronting a Life with Epilepsy

Stacia Kalinoski

 University of Minnesota Press
Minneapolis
London

Published by the University of Minnesota Press
111 Third Avenue South, Suite 290
Minneapolis, MN 55401-2520
http://www.upress.umn.edu

ISBN 978-1-5179-1746-3 (pb)

A Cataloging-in-Publication record for this book
is available from the Library of Congress.

Printed in the United States of America on acid-free paper

The University of Minnesota is an equal-opportunity
educator and employer.

34 33 32 31 30 29 28 27 26 25   10 9 8 7 6 5 4 3 2 1

Contents

Prologue // 1

1   You Can Run Faster // 5
2   Tonic-Clonic (or, How to Worry a Parent) // 14
3   Tough As Nails // 26
4   Cornhusker // 32
5   Sleepless in Seattle // 43
6   Calming the Storm // 53
7   Déjà Vu // 60
8   A Difficult Patient // 70
9   Missing Reminiscing // 76
10 Level 4: Denial // 86
11 Looking for Answers // 97
12 Bizarre and Unique // 110
13 Nowhere Else to Hide // 122
14 Jamais Vu // 130
15 Epilepsy Wins // 135
16 Termination // 142
17 The Best Place to Start Over // 146
18 Coming Home and Reaching New Heights // 153
19 Stigma, Up Close and Personal // 160
20 Black and White // 165
21 A Battery of Tests // 171

22 "You Are a Candidate" // 179

23 Back behind the Camera // 185

24 Brain Mapping // 194

25 Caregivers' Worry Never Ends // 209

26 *Brainstorm* // 216

Resources and Further Reading // 223

Acknowledgments // 227

Prologue

The earthy scent of soil and fresh rain filled my lungs as I powered on my watch, jogged up a short hill in my quiet Eugene neighborhood, and ran the mile-long stretch to jump onto the Amazon Trail. The name was fitting—rain kept the wood chips densely packed and the trees a bright, almost neon green this time of year, making spring perfect for marathon training in Oregon.

The 2011 Eugene Marathon was in May—just one month away—and I was in the best shape of my life, chasing a 2:50 marathon. A year earlier I had reached my goal of breaking 3:00 in Seattle, so now the plan was to chip away and eventually hit 2:43, the qualifying marker for the Olympic trials. I was nowhere near the caliber of Olympic athletes, but I'd have the chance to race with the best women in America if I progressed slowly and didn't get injured. For me, it was all about the chase, to find out how fast I could really run.

A soft mist started to fall as I finished my warm-up and geared up for my first 800-meter interval. Wiping the fog from my watch, I took a deep breath, hit the start button, and took off, my shoes kicking up mulch. The first interval felt good. I wish I could say the same about the next, but as my feet pounded the trail, the vivid green leaves of the trees started to blur slowly. I squeezed my eyes shut a few times in confusion, then in fear, as I glanced left and right. The familiar scenery ahead began to fade, like I was running into a cloud turning from white to gray. My pace slowed to a jog. The loop I ran almost daily suddenly looked foreign, as if I had turned a corner into a totally different city. The lefts and rights my feet normally took without even thinking were now dirt paths to nowhere. Trees that had once provided a scenic, comforting buffer from the streets were now barriers as I slowed down and tried to look beyond the mulch for any sense of direction toward home.

A few minutes later, I found myself standing on wet mulch, gazing at my surroundings. I was lost, confused, soaked, and nervous.

"Where am I?" I whispered aloud.

The trees stood silent.

The frightening experience slowly passed, but my confusion lingered. Anger started to build. Anger at my brain for failing me again. For failing me while I was doing something I loved. With no clue where to turn, I sat down on the trail and hoped my inner compass would somehow renavigate me. But my heart rate had yet to slow down, and as the emotions bubbled up, salty tears mixed with rain fell down my cheeks.

"Hey there, are you alright?"

A young couple in rain boots and umbrellas looked down at me, their eyes wide with concern. Wiping away my tears, I was equal parts embarrassed and grateful to see them.

"Hi, um, yes, I'm kind of lost," I replied, my voice shaky. "I was running and now I have no clue what part of the trail this is."

They asked for my address, and if they were surprised by my answer, they didn't show it. I was just two blocks from home.

They were nice enough to walk me to my door.

Before this run, I could always come up with an excuse to keep training and downplay the seriousness of my epilepsy. Over the last year, seizures had gradually started taking control of my life, but they hadn't directly interfered with the one thing that eased the stress of epilepsy—running—until now. Burning my shoulder on a hot iron, falling into a brick wall, breaking a tooth, and acquiring multiple black eyes were the ugly aftermath of a storm of neurons misfiring in my brain. But by the time those injuries had occurred, I had already lost consciousness.

That day on the trail was different. I had to physically, mentally, and emotionally endure a seizure that interrupted not only a challenging workout but also my sense of place and time, and it scared me.

The first part of the seizure that I consciously experienced is called an aura—a sensation of something to come; it's usually a warning that a larger seizure is on the way. Auras come in many forms, and this particular one is called "jamais vu," which means an unfamiliar feeling with something that's usually very familiar— like my running trail. On that day, the larger seizure struck when I lost awareness.

The aura from that day is ingrained in my memory. Most aren't though, and that's partly due to where in the brain my seizures were firing from. I struggle to recall other devastating seizures, only learning about them later from family, friends, and coworkers—or from lingering scars and bruises. If the seizures themselves weren't bad enough, having my memory escape me slowly and unwittingly began to take its toll. Leafing through the multiple scrapbooks I've created will evoke a range of emotions—from tears, to laughter, to surprise—but above all, I feel complete shock that the smile lighting up my eyes in photos with loved ones is a memory that has since escaped me forever.

As I gathered around a campfire recently with my siblings and parents, we opened up a game with some contemplative thought starters.

"Would you rather remember everything, bad or good? Or remember nothing?"

If only it was simple enough to be given a choice.

Gazing into the flames reminded me of all the firestorms that had ripped across my brain over the course of six years. Seizures had left behind bits and pieces, but the memories were often so fragmented that things fell out of context, and sometimes turned to ash.

Epilepsy can affect all types of memory. I struggle mostly with recalling events. For this book, I have relied heavily on close friends, family, medical records, and emails to fill in the blanks. Seizures have stolen many memories, both good and bad, from all points of my life. They have stormed through my highlight reels and my lowest moments, erasing some of the lessons that came with them. I'm often amazed when I think about how a brain so powerful—a conductor that directs every second of every movement, thought, and emotion—can also be so vulnerable when a storm passes through. The aftermath of those storms? Me, holding a scrapbook in my hands and struggling to recognize the girl in the photos.

While many experiences that shaped me have faded with each seizure, there's still so much I do recall. And when one particularly devastating seizure tore through my brain and upended my career, I was forced to dig deeper into my remaining memories—and the grit I developed as an athlete—to pick myself up and find the strength to take the biggest opportunity of my life.

1

You Can Run Faster

I ran. I ran on the icy snow-packed streets in my small Minnesota hometown as a teenager and on the rolling golf courses and tracks across the nation as a college athlete. I ran down long, flat roads in Nebraska, winding mulch trails in Oregon, and hills near my Michigan apartment as I relocated cities for my reporting career.

At the end of each day, running was always there. It was the one thing I could take with me wherever I went, a constant presence in a life filled with unpredictability. So many things kept me coming back every day to throw on a T-shirt and lace up my shoes. I ran to find energy and to release it; to shake off a bad mood or to lift a great one; to set goals or to accept not having met them; to set new limits and to test them; to explore my neighborhood and to get lost in it; to get places or to go nowhere; to try out new shoes, to wear out old ones; to see friends, to be alone, and to stay in shape. Running gave me clarity and took away stress.

A pair of new shoes every few months and a water fountain somewhere along my path were all I needed. Sports were my world growing up in Thief River Falls, Minnesota, a middle-class town of about eighty-eight hundred people tucked away in the northwest corner of the state. My first test in agility came in a pair of figure skates. A rainbow tutu, blush on my cheeks, and a bow in my hair completed my look for my town's annual winter ice show. After a few years in tights, it was clear I didn't have the poise and elegance to keep skating, but I was determined to be good at something, so I picked up a basketball.

My three younger siblings and I were expected to find a hobby to keep busy. One summer, my mom even called the local cable company to disconnect the TV, encouraging my sister, Sara, my identical twin brothers, Mike and Tom, and me to spend our time on sports and music. Mom was by no means a drill sergeant, nor did she expect us to be the best, but she wanted us to experience as much as possible. Don't like one sport? Try a new one! She set high standards for our family. A 5:00 a.m. alarm greeted her every morning for a long, brisk walk. As the director of the regional library system, she oversaw seven libraries in northwest Minnesota and was often on the road for meetings. From third to fifth grade, I'd head across the street to the library after school, drop off my coat and backpack in her office, and head over to a big chair by the large front windows and curl up with a book.

My dad, Greg, was calm, reliable, and pragmatic, a good balance for my mom's intensity. He worked as a farm business management instructor for our local community college, traveling to farms across the region to assist owners with their businesses. In the spring, he planted wheat and soybeans on land he had grown up on, an hour from Thief River Falls. My siblings and I spent some of our childhood summers running around the farm, driving the tractor and combine.

In middle school, sports took over. You could soon find me all year round with Sara and friends in pleated tennis skirts, basketball shorts, cloth running shorts, and T-shirts with the sleeves rolled up or cut off. Cute sports tops and spandex leggings were still a ways off. Sporting apparel of my childhood was baggy, and professional sports culture was huge. Tearaway pants were as common as jeans in school, and colorful Starter jackets filled the hallways in the winter. My parents were happy to add a basketball hoop in our driveway, and my siblings and I often extended our court into the alley behind our house to play HORSE or two-on-two.

Sara was the creative one in the family; she always had an art project in her hands. Mike was persistent and determined, much like me. Our brother Tom was the mellow one—still driven but without the intensity of Mike and me. We grew up loving the comradery of team sports and get-togethers with friends on weekends. But at night, after dinner or sports practice, we either headed out to our part-time job or navigated to our own space to do homework.

During the school year, we saw each other mostly on weekends or briefly during the week for dinner and at the breakfast table.

From middle school until the end of high school, my calendar year was divided into athletic seasons. Tennis in the fall, basketball in the winter, track in the spring, and camps and practice in the summer. On warm summer evenings, I'd strap on rollerblades, grab my tennis racket, and roll down the alley to meet my best friend, Kara. With huge, sky-blue eyes, Kara was extroverted to my introverted, spunky to my serious. We'd race to the nearby courts to practice, chatting nonstop. The summer sun stays up late in Minnesota, making up for the harsh winters. But the darkness that eventually took over never kept us from practicing. Kara and I discovered how to light up the night by "opening" the electrical circuit for the court lights. (Technically, we broke in.) When no one was free to play tennis with me, I got creative, practicing my returns against the garage door.

I loved the adrenaline rush those sports gave me, and many of my close friendships were formed during practices and on the road. Northwest Minnesota is mostly rural, so we'd often travel anywhere from 20 to 175 miles once or twice a week to compete against other teams. Many bus rides with my tennis teammates were nearly silent as we worked to finish homework before we competed, but they were often filled with laughter on the way home.

Tennis brought out my competitive spirit, although it didn't always come out in the best ways. My calf muscles turned solid black-and-blue in autumn from whacking my racket against them repeatedly in frustration if my serve strayed too far left or my return landed too deep. Tennis was my favorite challenge. The hardest thing about the sport wasn't the physical part—I could sprint up, down, and across that court all day. For me, it was the mental game. Every sport lends itself to lessons in mental toughness, and tennis was full of challenges. Missed shots and forced errors tested my mental readiness like nothing else.

I played a mix of varsity singles and doubles throughout high school and found the most success in doubles with Kara. She knew me better than anyone and kept me in line when she saw that I was getting worked up. Maybe she was able to do this because she was the youngest of four siblings. Kara had to learn to manage her three big brothers' personalities, whereas I, as the oldest of four, was the dominant personality at home. Kara and I met in grade school and navigated middle school and high school together. From piano recitals and tennis matches to first relationships and personal hardships, she has been a constant in my life. For everything we have in common, however, we couldn't be more different. But our dynamic worked well on the tennis court in our youth, and I would come to depend on her friendship in the hard times ahead.

While I absolutely loved competing in tennis and basketball, track became a bigger focus for me toward the end of high school. The track season started in mid-March, but we weren't quite able to leave the basketball gym just yet. Below-freezing temperatures often stick around until early spring in Minnesota, and the snow usually had no intention of stopping or melting in time to visit the track. In the first few weeks of the season, you could find our varsity group running stairs in the two-story gym, with lots of twists and turns through doors and around the wooden staircases. This whipped us into decent enough shape to compete at a couple indoor meets until the snow melted. The team was small but fun, with a mix of sprinters, mid-distance runners, throwers, and jumpers. Seventh grade was the start of many races around the oval, but it took time for me to find the right distance and understand my potential. My 400-meter time wasn't very competitive, and I grew discouraged when I didn't see my hard work pay off. I tried my luck at doubling the distance with the 800-meter run, but I wasn't satisfied.

You can run faster.

My coaches doubled the distance once more, and I laced up for the 1,600-meter run my junior year. I qualified for the state meet, and that first taste of success motivated me to start running that summer. By autumn of my senior year, I figured I could handle competing in cross country races in addition to tennis.

My 2002 debut race proved that even seniors can make embarrassing rookie mistakes. Mine took place on our home turf when I took a wrong turn on the golf course. A local newspaper photo captured my feelings perfectly. Poor form and the bewildered look on my face seemed to ask, "What the hell is this sport?" But to my surprise, I was the first girl to cross the finish line, so I laughed off the wrong move once I caught my breath. The 4K race was the hardest thing I'd ever done. The inclines were nothing like a track, and I had a strange, uneasy feeling not knowing how much farther the course was.

Juggling tennis matches and cross country training that season, I squeezed in three races to qualify for the Section 8 regional cross country meet. I outran another girl to the finish line by a scarce .32 seconds to grab the last qualifying spot for the Minnesota State Cross Country Championships. I was excited to compete at state, but once the gun went off and dozens of colorful jerseys bolted ahead, I got a reality check. I needed more miles on the pavement—hundreds more—to catch up. Nobody ran that fast up in my neck of the woods. Competing against the best in the state inspired me to train harder for the upcoming track season. That winter I set the alarm earlier for my paper route. My cloth newspaper bag was stained with ink from copies of the *Grand Forks Herald*. After dropping off the bag, I swapped my wet boots for dry running shoes and then pushed myself for an intense twenty to thirty minutes on the slippery roads.

My senior track season started off strong, and I was excited to receive a call from the University of Minnesota's track and cross country coach, Gary Wilson, inviting me to campus for a recruiting visit later that season. I had already been accepted, and the U's School of Journalism was my top choice, but I never expected track to enter the conversation. Wilson was a New Yorker with a friendly, sarcastic attitude that put me at ease right away. A handful of other track and cross country programs also showed interest.

My first race that year proved to me that my off-season training had paid off. I reached a personal record in the 1,600-meter run at our second meet of the season, breaking the high school record with a time of 5:09. Then I tried the 3,200-meter run and broke the school record. The success was the best validation. My race schedule was pretty consistent: two distance events at every track meet, usually twice a week. When I wasn't competing, I was in the weight room, pushing through heavy workouts to strengthen my legs. I was too inexperienced to know that so much racing, lifting, and intense training were hurting, not helping, me.

It didn't take long for my iliotibial band to flare up; the pain taught me how crucial that long band of fascia connecting my hip to my knee was to my running ability. It was my first real athletic injury. I got back in shape just in time to qualify for the state meet and was excited to make the trip with my good friend Erin, who had qualified in the 400-meter dash. I took sixth place in the 1,600-meter run and ninth place in the 3,200-meter run. Though my race times were disappointing, medaling at state was my proof that hard work can pay off, and that feeling would push me throughout my time at the University of Minnesota and beyond.

Three months after the state track meet would come my first introduction to the rigors of college cross country: intervals, tempo runs, long runs, and plenty of hills. That August, I drove the six hours from my hometown to the University of Minnesota campus, I met my new teammates, and then we headed up to the far northeast corner of Minnesota. Preseason cross country camp at Camp Voyageur in Ely would bring a mix of hard workouts, outside activities, great food, and fun games to bond with teammates.

I felt out of place at first because I had never been part of a distance team with training partners. I loved my small high school track team, made up of mostly sprinters. My college team, on the other hand, was filled with an abundance of high-mileage, experienced runners. Some of my teammates were averaging forty-five to fifty miles a week. My maximum weekly distance in high school was twenty-five miles, and my longest run was around six miles, which I soon realized was a joke at the collegiate level. I was a walk-on with a short cross country résumé who needed to log a lot more miles.

I also felt out of place for another reason—spandex and sports bras. The two pieces were the general, and only, practice attire. My high school team practiced in nylon or cotton shorts and T-shirts with the sleeves cut off or rolled back and tucked into our sports bra straps. I didn't even own spandex shorts. Getting comfortable in minimal clothing took a while.

After camp, I moved into freshmen dorms, where I was paired up with another freshman, Joellen. We had become friends immediately at camp; we were both about the same skill level with similar personalities, so we trained together often and were basically inseparable. Coach Wilson outlined workouts based on our abilities, grouping together women who ran about the same pace, so that we could push each other. Everything was based on our speed and strength. Those running fifty miles a week or more usually stuck together, while those with less experience stuck together at thirty to forty miles a week. The latter was my group, and they were fun to train with. Sunday long runs gave my body a new test of endurance.

Training with an entirely new group of women was both intimidating and exciting. They were fun and encouraging, yet competitive, making for perfect teammates.

My first collegiate race in the fall of 2003 was only the sixth cross country race of my life and my first ever 6K. The gun went off at the University of Minnesota Golf Course, my teammates bolted forward, and I soon got a wake-up call as to just how hard Division 1 cross country was going to be. Climbing damp, grassy hills while dodging twigs and wet leaves is challenging enough, but add in multiple athletes jockeying for position to stay within the race boundaries, and you end up with flying elbows and a good chance of tripping in the first mile.

That race was just a warm-up. One of the largest collegiate cross country meets in the country—the Roy Griak Invitational—came just two weeks later on the same course.

This time, hundreds of elbows were flying. A tiny bit of rain can turn portions of a golf course into an obstacle course. I settled right in the middle pack, trudging through patches of muddy grass that the lead runners kicked up with their spikes. Hills made this even more taxing, as my legs worked harder to lift my spikes out of the swampy ground on the incline. Though the descending hills ahead appeared to offer a break, the reality is that racing down a trail with hundreds of feet surrounding yours is a little scary. That's when the elbows really come out since every runner fears rolling an ankle.

We filled out a small journal each week where we documented daily miles, race recaps, and thoughts on how we were feeling. My entries were brief and to the point: "I get six to eight hours of sleep a night. I added another mile to my long run. I was happy with my performance last week." We brought our journals to practice every week for Wilson to look over while we trained, and he filled them with comments and returned them to us after practice. The journals tracked our progress to see if we were improving and served as a reference if we got injured or sick. If we felt run-down, Wilson usually directed us to get our iron level checked and eat a steak for dinner. I never got sick but felt run-down a lot, so I took iron supplements and ate meat every night. But writing about how I was feeling seemed unimportant if my times weren't improving.

Distance running, like any sport, rewards those who dedicate their time to improving. For a competitive and dedicated athlete, it was tough to realize that no matter how many miles I put in, I'd never catch up to some of my teammates. The only option was to push myself to continuously top my own personal bests. I listened to my coach, trained as hard as I could, and made some improvements. At the end of my freshman season, I received the "Blue Collar Award," my coach's term for the hardest worker.

My sophomore track season started well, as I shaved about fifteen seconds off a high school personal record. There's no better feeling than achieving a personal best. The indoor 3,000-meter run was replaced with the 3,000-meter steeplechase, an obstacle race to test endurance and mental toughness over the course of seven and a half laps. Five barriers, including a water pit, lay ahead for each lap. Barriers are much larger and sturdier than hurdles; they don't fall down. I'd never hurdled over anything before, but I learned the basics at practice along with a teammate as we prepared for our first race at Duke University.

On race day I lined up next to her and took a huge breath. The first steeple barrier loomed ahead, and the gun went off. Experienced athletes can hurdle each barrier, but as a novice I focused on solely jumping on them rather than over them. Then came the twelve-foot water pit. The goal was to jump onto the steeple with one foot and as far out as I could with the other to avoid falling. It's a test of strength, balance, and, most of all, fearlessness. I pushed myself, but the water pit won twice in that race after I stumbled over the barrier, leaving me drenched and discouraged.

When a sports reporter covering the event for the University of Minnesota's student-run newspaper approached me with questions, I gave a light-hearted response: "For me, it can only get better."

Making fun of situations I clearly suck at usually helps me move on. I'm not one to quit after one failure, so I picked myself up out of the water jump and ran the steeplechase again at another meet. But I approached each water jump more timidly to avoid falling and thus didn't improve. Steeples weren't for me.

My coach understood that not all of us would become All-Americans. He encouraged every runner, no matter where we finished in the pack, as long as we competed. He knew what we were capable of and reminded us that there's a difference between racing and competing. So here I was in August 2005, a few weeks from the start of my junior year, in the best shape of my life and feeling healthy both physically and mentally. Kara and I had recently returned from a backpacking trip through Europe, and our adventures were all I could think about. But one Tuesday night in early August my health took a completely unexpected turn.

2

Tonic-Clonic (or, How to Worry a Parent)

Insomnia had crept into my life over the last year. Sleeping pills provided some relief but not enough. This made my summer training workouts even tougher than they already were, but I kept plugging away because cross country camp was coming up. That early August afternoon in 2005, I was working one of my summer jobs at the alumni center and messaged my boyfriend at the time, Chris.

"I'm about to fall asleep at work because I took sleeping pills this morning and I keep on dozing off . . ."

After work, I jumped on my bike and sped off to my apartment off campus, which I shared with two track teammates, Christine and Vanessa, and my high school friend Brittany. Later that evening, we said our good nights and headed for bed. I climbed to the top of the bunk in the room I shared with Brittany and tried to fall asleep. Nothing felt out of the ordinary as I eventually nodded off. Life was good.

A few hours of peaceful sleep were all any of us would get that night. Around two o'clock in the morning, my roommates woke up to me yelling loudly. Christine jumped out of bed and raced to my room.

"I assumed you may have found a spider in your bed or something silly, but I found you face down in your pillow convulsing," she recalled. "I carefully rolled you to your side and noticed that there was quite a bit of blood on the sheets that appeared to have come from your mouth."

I had bitten my tongue, which isn't uncommon in tonic-clonic seizures. Unconscious, I had no clue I was convulsing or screaming and couldn't imagine how terrifying it must have been for my roommates. Christine cared for a girl who had seizures, so she knew a seizure when she saw one. Paramedics rushed in to help me outside and onto the waiting stretcher. The intense glare of the hospital lights blinded me as the ambulance pulled up to the emergency room at the University of Minnesota Medical Center. My one memory of the entire night is a snapshot of getting out of the ambulance.

The doctor performed a neurological assessment and ordered a CT scan to rule out a brain bleed or a tumor. Tumors can cause seizures, and thankfully my scan was clear of trouble. The clean scan was reassuring, so now I was more curious than anxious. The doctor didn't find a tumor or anything else that required immediate hospitalization.

How worried should I be?

I was released with instructions to follow up with a neurologist the following week. By this point it was going on four o'clock in the morning. I was too fatigued and confused by what had just unfolded to be afraid or to process the unexpected night, let alone call my parents. They would only panic, barrage me with questions, and jump in the car to come down. The only thing I wanted at that moment was to sleep for two days. I don't remember how I got home, but I headed straight for my bedroom, then stopped and looked wearily up toward the top bunk. Tonight, it was either my comfy bed, a lumpy couch, or the hard floor. My body ached for comfort, so I took a few anxious steps toward the wooden ladder and slowly climbed up. My hands shook as they grabbed each step, but fatigue silenced my inner conscience. It was surely saying:

Why the hell would you climb up to a bunk bed? You just had an awful seizure!

Brain fog can push aside good judgment.

You didn't fall out. You'll be fine.

I reached the top and climbed into bed, too tired to see straight anymore. But the dried blood on my pillow couldn't be missed. I grimaced at the sight and flipped the pillow over.

Ugh. What made me bleed?

Exhaustion overwhelmed me, and I assumed my brain would

fall into a deep sleep after everything it had gone through that night. But once I hit the pillow and closed my eyes, the room started spinning.

I wondered if this was the start of another seizure. Every muscle in my body tensed in anticipation, and I held my breath until the point of passing out. Unable to take the suspense, I forced my eyes open. The room was still spinning. Colors of purple, blue, and yellow spun like a tornado across the room. A wave of nausea spread over me, powerful enough to overcome the fear of a seizure. I passed out into a deep sleep.

I was greeted the next morning with a headache, then a groggy playback of the night before. Only one thought consumed me.

Why did I have a seizure?

I racked my brain: I was young, healthy, and had never had a concussion. Heck, I'd never even had the flu, a fever, mononucleosis, or any other common ailment in my lifetime, and I had grown up in the 1990s, well before kids started getting flu shots. My siblings and parents stayed healthy too, enough so that over the course of twenty-three years raising us, my parents never missed work due to sick kids. There must have been something in the water in Thief River Falls.

No one in my family or extended family had ever had a seizure.

So why did a seizure strike so unexpectedly?

Do seizures affect running?

Wait. Shoot!

I grabbed a calendar. It was Wednesday. My head dropped. I was supposed to do a workout today. But even the idea of my body in motion, my arms swinging and head bobbing, made my head spin.

Ugh, please body, recover by tomorrow.

As much as I wanted an answer in that moment, I realized that overthinking something that only doctors could explain was a waste of time. Why dwell on it?

I had to call my mom and dad.

My parents would worry, understandably, but that's the last thing I wanted. It would turn into constant check-ins to see how I was doing. Of all the things my parents could worry about with two daughters now in college, a random seizure had to be the last thing to cross their minds. I dialed my mom's number, and my throat tightened in anticipation. She answered in her usual cheery tone but also with a note of surprise.

"Hi Stacia! I never get a call from you at this time. Do you not work today?"

I steadied my voice to prevent it from cracking.

"Hi, Mom. No, I'm at home," I said calmly. "Something really weird happened last night. I . . . had a seizure." I forced the last three words out, my voice clipping at the end. My mom gasped.

"Stacia! What?!"

The shock in her voice forced me to sit down and take a deep breath.

"How?? Why??" she asked in a frantic whisper. I could picture her, one hand pressed to her mouth, leaning back into her office chair.

"It was a grand mal. My roommates saw me convulsing into my pillow," I said, trying to minimize the uneasiness in my voice.

Grand mal was the extent of my knowledge of epilepsy. The medical term is "tonic-clonic." But what about the screaming? Is that common with a seizure? Unsure, I left that part out, as well as the blood.

"I'm sorry to worry you," I said quickly. "But things are OK. Christine called 911 and my roommates were there to help. The doctor did a CT scan, nothing concerning showed up—"

"Where did this come from?" she interrupted, trying not to sound too anxious. But she was too focused on the word "seizure" to concentrate on what I said next.

"I'm not sure, but the other tests they did were normal, so they released me relatively quickly last night," I replied, slowing down my words to calm her down. "I'm going to see a neurologist soon."

"OK, OK," she said, trying to collect her thoughts. Mom was familiar with epilepsy; she had witnessed one of her employees at the library have this type of seizure twice before.

"I'll talk to your dad and decide when to come down."

"No, it's OK. There's no point until I see the doctor, and I'll tell you what he says," I reassured her.

My parents lived six hours north, worked full-time, and had my high school brothers to take care of. I had always been very independent, and I told her it wasn't necessary to come all the way down for a thirty-minute doctor's appointment. My mom disagreed.

The lack of clarity about the seizure was unsettling for my mom. Different scenarios swirled in her mind. Had something happened in my childhood that she wasn't aware of? Maybe at daycare? Had I hit my head at some point? There were so many questions that had no answers. Researching epilepsy was difficult; at the time, there was limited information available online. My mom relied on articles from university libraries, but they didn't fill her thirst for knowledge the way talking to a physician could. Her employee's epilepsy provided some experience with handling a seizure, but not the understanding of what this would mean going forward. My mom would attend all my appointments and relay the information to my dad, who stayed home with my brothers. Seizures were unfamiliar to him, too, but he put his faith in doctors. The sense of calm in his voice when calling to check in helped to offset the tension in my mom's.

"We have to trust today's medical care and move forward," he would say.

Trust over worry seemed more logical and less stressful, so I tried to adopt the same mindset. More than anything, I was curious. What causes a young, well-functioning brain to abruptly change course?

Leading up to the neurology appointment, running offered a welcome distraction. But one question kept popping up throughout the week. Would the doctor tell me to stop training? Once I climbed into bed each night there was nothing to distract my mind from racing, so I'd stare at the ceiling, fearing that the bright lights of a hospital entrance would greet me again at 2:00 a.m. When the alarm jolted me awake each morning, I sighed in relief to feel my comforter against my skin.

My mom drove down for the appointment a day early. She

needed to see the Emergency Department entrance for herself to absorb what had happened in her own way. The seizure consumed her thoughts the entire six-hour drive, and she gripped the wheel as she approached the university. White-knuckled, she turned onto the sprawling green campus to see students my age strolling down the sidewalks, biking, and laughing as they took in the last few weeks of freedom and beautiful weather before the fall semester started. The sight left her bewildered that just a week earlier, I had been one of those carefree students.

Now my mom needed to understand why her twenty-year-old daughter had wound up in the hospital. The bright red "Emergency" signage caught her eye on the busy road, and she slowed down and pulled into the entrance. The doors slid open as a few nurses walked outside in their scrubs. She put the car in park and squinted through her window at the doors as they opened and closed, observing each doctor and nurse coming and going. The sight calmed her somewhat, helping her come to terms with what I faced in the ER and prepare herself for what was to come.

She left the hospital to pick me up, and I jumped in the car with a bright hello, only to see her usual smile replaced with a worried look. My heart sank. I reached over and gave her a reassuring hug.

"Thanks for driving me! Don't worry, Mom, everything is going to be fine. The doctor didn't find a tumor."

I figured cancer would have been the worst-case scenario, and since the hospital had sent me home the night of the seizure, the upcoming testing wouldn't reveal anything earth-shattering. Without a medical degree, patients can either go down a rabbit hole of fearing the worst or believe they're invincible. I realized it was best to wait and see what the doctor said. My brain was too complex for me to even begin to understand all the things that could be wrong with it.

After a short drive, we arrived at the medical school to meet neurologist Dr. Miguel Fiol, who would perform my first electro-encephalogram (EEG). I was about to get a crash course in epilepsy and the science of the brain. Dr. Fiol explained that an EEG measures brain waves to look for spikes, which can signal a surge of electrical activity. Epileptic seizures are caused by an excessive amount of electrical activity in one or more parts of the brain that interrupts normal brain signals.

The brain holds billions of nerve cells that produce tiny electrical signals, and they form patterns called brain waves. These waves travel via an electrical current through the central nervous system, sending constant messages to other parts of the body. In a healthy brain, neurons fire in a consistent pattern. But multiple things can cause those neurons to misfire, causing a seizure. Anyone can have a seizure at any point in their lives, and it won't necessarily mean they have epilepsy. Toxicity from illicit drugs like cocaine and heroin, withdrawal from dependence on alcohol, and high fevers in children can all provoke a seizure. The latter is called a febrile seizure. Sudden drops in blood pressure and very low or high blood sugar can also provoke seizures because of the unexpected shift in the blood supply to the brain or in the brain's sugar levels. Unless provoking factors go unresolved or continue to reoccur, these seizures usually are one-time events.

Stroke, traumatic brain injury, and brain infections like meningitis and encephalitis can also provoke a seizure, and they can all eventually lead to epilepsy in some people. The injury or infection can kill nerve cells and leave behind an area of damaged tissue called a lesion. Over time, this scar tissue can disrupt the brain's electrical activity, causing nerve cells to misfire, sparking a huge surge of electrical activity. This is an epileptic seizure. More than two unprovoked seizures indicate epilepsy.

In my case, a tumor was ruled out, as were other potential provoking factors. That was a good start. Dr. Fiol hoped the EEG could give us some answers. The EEG is also used to rule out another type of seizure, called psychogenic. Psychogenic non-epileptic seizures (PNES) are caused not by an electrical disturbance in the brain but rather by a physical reaction to psychological stress. They are often called stress seizures. One doctor told me it's like a seizure happens instead of a panic attack. People with PNES don't have control over their actions during a seizure, similar to people with epilepsy.

I wasn't experiencing any type of psychological stress and I didn't have another seizure prior to the appointment, so an EEG was the only way to find out what was wrong. A friendly EEG technician separated my hair in various spots and attached electrodes—quarter-shaped sticky metal disks—to my scalp and forehead. The electrodes connected to wires that connected to an EEG machine that would detect any unusual spikes in the brain waves. My first EEG lasted twenty-two minutes. The result was mildly abnormal, with some slower than normal brain wave frequency in my right temporal lobe. But there wasn't clear-cut evidence for epileptic activity.

OK, good! Everything is going to be fine!

Then I was told an EEG measures just a small amount of brain activity at one point in time, so it was not possible to rule epilepsy out. My heart sank.

I might have epilepsy? Me?

Dr. Fiol scheduled a sleep-deprived EEG next, saying that some people usually only have seizures in their sleep. I nodded, then stopped.

My first seizure had happened in my sleep. If that happened again, then what? Would Dr. Fiol restrict my class load or track workouts?

I shut out all thoughts of the seizure and quickly transitioned back into college life.

The cross country season was getting underway, and I was relieved that the seizure turned out to be just a minor interruption.

But two weeks later came another interruption, this time during an afternoon nap, with no one there to witness it. I awoke to a blurry view of a bunk bed far above my head, throbbing in my left eye and cheekbone, and a crick in my neck. My arm trembled as I reached my hand behind my neck, only to find a hard surface.

Why am I on the floor?

I twisted my neck in search of an answer, wincing in pain as I came eye to eye with the bottom of a desk.

The room, the desk, every square inch of space looked unfamiliar.

Dazed, I rolled over to squint back up at the bunk bed. It looked a mile high. Just then, a flashback to a bloody pillow. My throat went dry, and I looked back up to the ceiling. *Is that my bed?* My gaze wandered to the ladder, and I stared for what seemed like an eternity before my brain matched the grains in the wood and number of steps in front of me. Now I could picture myself grabbing the sides with ease and jumping up onto the mattress. There was no railing. Then it registered. I lifted my hand to the left side of the growing lump on my left cheek and tender eye, then looked up to the pillow and back down to the floor. Directly in the path was the desk, positioned perpendicular to the bunk beds. My stomach dropped.

I looked up at the bed, down to the desk, and back again about four times. My face would had to have collided with the sharp corner of the desk on the way down. There was no other path. I drew in a shallow breath and shuffled over to the mirror. A huge cut directly over the corner of my eye stared back at me. An ugly bruise of blue and purple masked the swelling already underway over my eye and on the left side of my face.

Either I had had another seizure, or I had fallen out of bed and then suffered a concussion. The former was probably the truth, though I didn't want to admit it. Or had a seizure also caused a concussion when I hit the floor? I knew it would be impossible to hide what had happened.

"Wait! What time is it??" I suddenly panicked. "No, wait! What day is it? Am I supposed to be somewhere??"

There was no one there to answer me.

My face burned as I jumped up and ran across the room to grab my cross country journal.

Could that give me the date? I ripped it open to find my last entry—a four-mile recovery run yesterday. Today's page was blank for mileage, but a team meeting was penned in for that afternoon.

"Shoot," I muttered, leaning against the wall. "What awful timing. I can't miss a team meeting."

There was enough time to ice my cheek, so I rummaged through the freezer and spotted a bag of vegetables. Good enough. The bag was already burning my fingers, and I dreaded how it would feel. I wrapped it in a paper towel, placed it against my face with one hand, and then gingerly pressed the frozen bag over my face and eye.

I flinched, but knowing the ice would slow the swelling, I sat down in the kitchen and timed myself. Ten minutes later I gently pulled the ice pack off my face, wincing at the cold burn. I tossed the veggies back in the freezer, patted some concealer on my face, headed out the door, and jumped on my bike. I dreaded the inevitable questions. Christine was one of the first to notice the black eye under my makeup.

The seizure and possible concussion left me with no memory of that meeting or what my coach or teammates might have said.

The timing was perfect for a sleep-deprived EEG. EEGs aren't always helpful unless patients actually have a seizure during the monitoring. Because of this, doctors sometimes try to provoke one. This time he ordered me to stay up all night before the appointment. Sleep deprivation can make people with epilepsy more prone to having seizures.

My recent insomnia made it easy to stay up very late, but all night? I wasn't a coffee drinker, and I rarely drank soda. Books and movies would put me to sleep fast, so how could this work? A friend volunteered to stay up with me. Diet Coke stretched my threshold even longer. My eyelids began to droop just before the sun started to rise, but my mom arrived in time to get me up and moving before the appointment.

The EEG that morning recorded my brain for forty-one minutes and evaluated my brain activity while I was awake, drowsy, and asleep. This time, Dr. Fiol shared that the results appeared normal. My tense shoulders sank into my chair as I finally relaxed.

This EEG didn't show anything concerning. Neither did a CT scan.

But he reminded me again that a normal EEG doesn't rule out epilepsy. He ordered an MRI and started me on an antiseizure medication called Keppra.

I hesitated. Brain medication? I worried that I would feel weird, that it would affect my schoolwork and running. Still, I reasoned it's probably better than having another seizure. Maybe I have epilepsy, maybe I don't, but if so, medication will take care of it. End of story.

He also started me on a sleep medication. I got up to leave.

"Hold on," he said.

Unfortunately, medication didn't take care of Dr. Fiol's other concern. My heart had been monitored during the EEG and was found to be beating very slowly with occasional extra beats.

"I want you to see a cardiologist and to get an EKG."

Just like an electroencephalogram records the brain's electrical system, an electrocardiogram (EKG) records the heart's electrical system.

The MRI of my brain done the following day didn't show anything concerning.

One week later, I hopped on my bike to get the EKG. My route to the medical school was a straight shot from my apartment, and I felt lucky that all my problems could be dealt with on campus.

At the EKG appointment a technician placed electrodes on my chest to detect the strength and timing of the electrical signals that caused my heart to beat. Mine was found to be doing what Dr. Fiol had noticed earlier, beating in the low 30s beats per minute (bpm). That's on the very low end for an athlete, which is usually between 40 and 60 bpm. Anything that falls below 60 bpm is diagnosed as bradycardia—a slower than normal heart rate.

My heart rate had always been slow, which doctors throughout my life had told me wasn't worrisome because I played sports. When someone is in shape, the heart doesn't need to work as hard to pump blood to organs. But if the heart pumps too slowly, less oxygen-rich blood flows to the body. This can cause someone to faint, which may mimic some types of seizures.

The cardiologist also ordered a Holter heart rate study. For forty-seven hours, I would go about my usual routine as a college student with a small device hanging from my neck and directly over my heart to record every activity I did, big or small, in a diary. My heart was averaging 55 bpm over the course of a day, maxing at 132 bpm while running and settling down at 31 bpm at rest. But it wasn't just slow at rest; it had abnormal rhythms. My heart was either skipping beats or producing extra heartbeats.

Why was my heart out of whack? Had it always had an irregular rhythm? Was it causing seizures? Or were seizures causing the heart issue?

Research has shown a connection between seizures and heart arrhythmias.

For now, I was asymptomatic. I hadn't been dizzy or hadn't fainted from the slow heart rate, so my doctor allowed me to keep working out.

Keppra didn't last long. The antiseizure medication gave me mood swings—a common side effect—so I stopped taking it after a month. The seizures didn't return after going off Keppra, so I optimistically believed the situation was behind me. I was confident that my health would be smooth sailing from there on out if I followed a few basic rules: exercise, sleep, and fruits and veggies.

3

Tough As Nails

Smooth sailing was not the path my feet took. A foot injury sidelined me for most of my junior track season. The pool and a bike became my new training ground, along with some other teammates who were in the same boat. We strapped a blue floating device to our backs, stepped into the pool, and started aqua jogging. The goal was to try and stay in shape by doing intervals. We jogged as quickly as we could for a minute or more, slowed down to an easy pace, and repeated this over and over. Increasing my heart rate was much harder in a pool. But running in place gave me time to think. The track made me physically stronger, but the pool toughened me mentally.

Rebounding from injuries takes rehabilitation, resilience, and resistance to the discouragement and doubt that creep into athletes' minds. Like many of my teammates, I was driven and sometimes stubborn, so accepting that injuries required a combination of downtime and a slow progression of strengthening and cross-training was frustrating.

Don't give up on yourself, Stacia.

As I focused on healing my foot, the seizures became a distant memory for me, but not for Christine. She noticed instances where I would blank out or not seem to be paying attention for five to ten seconds. Following this, she said, I would seem confused about the conversation we were having prior to the strange episodes.

I have no memory of experiencing those feelings, and it was embarrassing to hear of my close friend's perception. If those episodes were in fact seizures or something heart related, we never would have guessed. Seizures seemed pretty cut and dry to me at that point—you're either convulsing or you're not. I did not yet understand they can take on many different forms. After some time, Christine said she didn't notice the confusion anymore.

I rebounded from my foot injury by my senior year of cross country season and won the team's "Tough as Nails Award." The award symbolized mental toughness and commitment to the sport. "I never had to get in your face or yell at you because you always gave 100 percent," my coach recalled.

But the qualities that pushed me to reach personal goals were also the same qualities that hindered me at crucial moments with my health later on. Sudden problems with the brain and the heart don't always just go away, regardless of how minor they may seem. At twenty years old, though, I put my health problems in the rearview mirror and refocused on bigger things: my career.

My love of sports stuck with me on and off the track, dating back to high school. Devouring the sports section of the *Grand Forks Herald* with breakfast and catching the sports coverage on the local news before dinner sparked a career interest: sports reporting.

Talking into a microphone was already second nature. In my parochial elementary school, I wasn't shy about speaking in front of a crowd after being given the chance to do the scripture readings at our weekly mass. In high school, my mom noticed my enthusiasm for the local news and suggested I talk to Pat Sweeney, the sports director at WDAZ in Grand Forks, North Dakota, who'd been covering sports in the region for decades. He agreed to an interview for my school career project, and I put on my reporter hat and prepared a list of detailed questions. Pat was generous with his time and gave me a tour of the studio. I wrote detailed notes, but today I don't remember anything from our meeting other than that he sold me on the career. I wanted to be a reporter.

I also applied for an internship at my local AM radio station in town. The general manager took a chance on me, and when I showed up at KTRF on the first day and opened the door to the broadcast room, I looked over the huge soundboard with rows of colored buttons. The large microphone and a stack of papers with news headlines both excited and terrified me. I was inexperienced, unprepared, and intimidated. In no time I would be responsible for sharing community service announcements, news, and weather updates during the syndicated music shows. In Minnesota, the weather often *is* the news, so my job started with blizzard warnings from December into March.

By spring, the Minnesota Twins were in action. I'd interrupt the sportscast for ten seconds at the top of each hour to give the station identification. Twins fans across northwest Minnesota would hear a brief second of silence before I took a big breath and flipped the on-air switch:

"You're listening to the Minnesota Twins on AM 1230, KTRF in Thief River Falls."

My pitch was no doubt a little too high at first, but after a few games my vocal cords started to relax. My goal was to just sound as normal, and professional, as possible. I figured if they let me stay on the air, I couldn't have been terrible. My dad was my biggest fan, tuning in to every Twins game to listen for my short update each hour, and he didn't even follow baseball.

"You sounded very professional!" he would tell me when I got home. A little compliment, even from my dad, gave me enough confidence to stay on-air. My parents weren't the type to sugarcoat something if my siblings and I truly sucked at it, so I took the compliments at face value. At seventeen, my career path was set. All I knew was that I enjoyed the feeling of putting on the headphones, hitting the on-air switch, and broadcasting into that radio microphone. I wanted to shoot and edit video, too, so I would go the broadcast television route.

The TV news reporting courses I took at the University of Minnesota cemented my interest in this career path even further. A lot of time has passed since college, and a lot has happened since then. Epilepsy makes it difficult to recall what my classrooms looked like. I don't remember more than three of my classmates' names. But a handful of rules from my journalism classes that instructor Ken Stone drilled into our heads did stick with me.

"Find a personal angle to go with the story."

"White balance!"

Video cameras have a little switch you flip while holding up a piece of white paper to the lens. This makes sure that the color white stays white; otherwise all the video will show up with a different color temperature that doesn't look natural. Editing color is not the best use of time on a deadline. But Ken stressed one thing that was even more important.

"Check your audio levels on the camera during interviews, AND WEAR HEADPHONES! Your news director won't care if your video turns out blue as much as he will care about your botched audio." Video can usually be color corrected or replaced with other video. But most audio is very difficult to fix.

Ken became a huge mentor throughout my TV career with his honesty, knowledge, and support—always willing to look at my résumé tape even after college. He taught me to really listen to the people I interviewed.

After interning at WCCO in Minneapolis, I was fortunate to get an internship at a competitor across town, KSTP, under the tutelage of political reporter Tom Hauser. I spent all my time at the Minnesota State Capitol, cramped in a small office transcribing audio from the legislative sessions. It was my first taste of politics, and listening to lawmakers debate bills for hours gave me more respect for their role in shaping policy, though I knew this definitely wasn't the reporting path for me. Still, understanding that state and local government issues would be on my plate as a reporter, I eagerly took in the experience.

During my job search, my goal was to leave Minnesota but to stay in the Midwest, so I sent out a handful of tapes with no idea of what to expect. There are more than two hundred television markets in the United States, and most reporters start out in small markets, like Fargo, Sioux Falls, or Missoula. I wondered how many people would apply to the same stations as I was. Competition was intense, and I was competing with classmates and other college graduates near and far. The realization made my heart thump. I drew in a large breath as scenarios swirled through my mind.

What kind of stories are on their résumé tapes? Do they shoot and edit better than I do? Do their voices sound more professional?

Thankfully, I didn't have to wait long to find out. Not long after graduation, a news director at the ABC affiliate KHGI-TV in Kearney, Nebraska, was the first to offer me a job. I'd be a bureau reporter in Grand Island, a city of about fifty thousand people.

Even though I had spent the last two years working for this moment, getting an actual job offer outside of Minnesota was still a surprise.

I eagerly accepted the position; I didn't have the patience to wait for another potential offer. Moving out of state would get me out of my comfort zone, forcing me to meet new people with different views from my own. That was crucial if I wanted to be an unbiased reporter. My parents shared my excitement when I called, with a tone of relief in their voices. I had something to show for my four-year college education, and for that we were all grateful.

In the spring of 2007, my friends and I threw our commencement hats into the air. By July, I had packed up my apartment, shared a goodbye toast with my college friends, and driven off to the Cornhusker State. Reality didn't set in until I crossed into Iowa and looked back at Minnesota in the rearview mirror. A track meet in Lincoln had been my first trip to Nebraska, and now I'd be a resident there.

Soon everything I'd learned in college—gathering facts and information and shooting, writing, and editing a story every night—would be on a strict deadline. A mix of enthusiasm and hesitation filled my thoughts. My college journalism instructor had once been a reporter and anchor himself, and he had been my only real judge. Now, my work would be in the hands of experienced anchors and producers, and I'd have to get used to taking criticism very quickly. Hair and makeup would be in my own hands, a task I already disliked. A ponytail had framed my face for 90 percent of my life as an athlete, and I didn't want to start teasing and curling my hair. That would be inevitable though to look professional. So would putting on lipstick, which had always felt silly on me.

What I didn't yet know was that aside from producing my own stories, I'd be responsible for sending them to Kearney via satellite and setting up my own live shots—like a glorified selfie with a really heavy video camera. The countdown would start right when I opened the bureau front door at 2:00 p.m., and all this had to happen within eight hours in order to go live on the 10:00 p.m. newscast. I took a big breath and leaned back into the seat of my car, turned on the radio, and glanced out the window. Nothing but wide-open fields ahead of me, a reassuring sight.

The possibility of having another seizure never crossed my mind. Junior year felt like a distant memory now. The reason for those seizures would always remain a mystery, and I was OK with that. I left that part of my life in Minneapolis. I wouldn't find out until years later that some seizures don't have any symptoms at all.

4

Cornhusker

The KHGI-TV News logo caught my eye as I slowly ventured into downtown Grand Island, Nebraska, for my first day of work. It was July 2007. I parked my car and looked into the storefront window with butterflies in my stomach.

Here we go.

I felt pretty good about my writing, shooting, and editing abilities as I stepped into the news bureau. Steve White, a seasoned journalist and the bureau's chief reporter, greeted me with a firm welcoming handshake. He was helpful and friendly from the start. We chatted on the way back to my new desk, and I quickly realized there would be a lot to learn once my eyes landed on the huge, intimidating video camera. I swallowed hard. This job was not going to be easy.

My stomach tightened as I picked up the camera, and I nearly dropped it. Compared to my camera from college, this was like a small suitcase, the kind of weight you have to lift with your legs, not your back. Thankfully I was strong enough to lift the camera and keep it steady on my right shoulder. I moved my hand to the side of the camera and gently pressed it. A small cassette tape popped out. Steve brought me over to the editing room. Inside I found a bulky TV monitor, two VCRs, and a huge editing deck with tons of computer keys in different sizes and colors scattered about. It was about the size of a Mac desktop but five times the width, and it looked ancient.

What the heck is that?

What does the JOG key do? What does that even mean?

Steve was about to give me a lesson in linear editing, also called tape-to-tape editing—a TV technology from the 1950s. In college, I had learned nonlinear editing on a digital timeline, and the methods were polar opposite. He got me through the first few weeks, and I was grateful for his help. But soon I was on my own. For the 10:00 p.m. newscast, I was the only person in the bureau to write the story, edit it, send it to the station, and then set up my live shot. I had always been independent, but this was a crash course in self-sufficiency and quick problem solving.

One night early on at the station, in a time crunch after covering a city council meeting, I pressed a wrong button while editing and had to fix the mistake on the fly. Not long after, I mixed up the audio channels, switching my voice track with that of the interviewee.

Shit! Yikes, figure it out!

That story barely made it on the air. Mistakes, major or minor, stole time away from editing a solid story.

My lesson in double-checking facts involved the one thing a reporter shouldn't mess up in the Cornhusker State—corn. Agriculture is huge in Nebraska. I enjoyed interviewing farmers, and I knew enough about farming to ask the right questions. Just mentioning that my dad worked in agriculture management sparked an instant connection. Because of this, I looked forward to covering one of the state's biggest events, Husker Harvest Days.

I called my dad that fall day while writing my story and referenced a specific part of a new combine. He stopped me halfway through the script.

"You were going to call the front of the combine a twelve-row corn picker!" he told me, laughing. "It's a twelve-row corn header." I now have no memory of that story or the call, but Nebraska farmers would have never forgiven me.

Details, details.

Facts aside, the most challenging part of being a newbie was grasping how many issues were on city council and school board agendas and figuring out which topics were the most important to cover. I needed to learn the politics of the city and the county, and though Steve was a huge help, there was no better way to do that than by attending those long, dry meetings. As a nightside reporter, this would be my beat. Figuring out what I should or shouldn't pack into a news story could be overwhelming. In journalism, reporters are told to find the meat of the story and discard all the fat. Cutting things down to ninety seconds was tough because I assumed viewers should know about everything that happened at a meeting. But TV news is not meant to detail every fact. Finding a simple but compelling focus amid a pile of meeting notes is the difficult part. My ears were tuned for good sound bites, but everything about the city budget seemed newsworthy.

My Minnesota accent was thick, and I was told to fix my long *o* and long *a* sounds. I didn't know my dialect sounded odd in Nebraska, but the anchors sure did. One night I got a phone call to revoice my story to change a few words. Reporters and anchors in large media markets train themselves to ditch their regional accents for one called "General America," the accent you hear from broadcasters and actors. It's comparable to parts of the Midwest (Chicago) and the West Coast. For example, the short *a* for apple is the same *a* for bag. Minnesotans tend to say "bag" with a long *a*. Your voice should provide no clue that you're from the Northeast, the Deep South, or the Upper Midwest, unless you report for a local station in your area.

I listened closely to the dialect and caught myself when voicing a story. Yep, definitely sounded Minnesoootan! I would usually revoice a few times. Once I had a good grasp on shooting video, editing, writing, and talking with a neutral TV voice, I knew reporting was a great career for me. The opportunity to meet new people and tell their stories, along with the creative aspect of the job, made me happy to come to work every day.

July 4, 2008, made me even happier. On that beautiful, cloudless afternoon, I remember looking up at a B-17 Flying Fortress with awe. It's not every day a news reporter gets to ride in a World War II bomber, much less a rookie reporter like me, but I was about to get that chance.

Still, I can only remember this event by piecing details together like a news story. A photograph showing me interviewing the pilot and crew is all I have to remind me of that day. It's amazing how a single photo can bring some events and feelings back to life—even for just a few seconds. It's like seeing the DVD cover of a romantic comedy you haven't watched in twenty years and then recalling one brief scene. Just like reading a synopsis of the movie likely brings more details back, reading my news report from that day helps a few details resurface.

A crew that was doing a multicity tour with the airplane stopped at the Central Nebraska Regional Airport in Grand Island that Friday, and I was lucky enough to cover the story. I lifted the heavy camera onto my shoulder, did a few interviews, chatted with the crew, took video of the plane, and prepared to leave. But the pilot casually asked if I wanted a ride. I looked at him in surprise.

"Really, me??"

"Absolutely!" he nodded, grinning.

I grabbed my camera and followed the pilot up the stairs and into the plane. The bomb bays were the first thing to catch my attention. Complete destruction would have been dropped right below my feet multiple times. The gravity of that reality startled me.

"Whoa!" is all I could say, looking down. The word spoke for so many thoughts running through my head, namely, gratitude for our American soldiers. Each bomber typically had a crew of ten men.

I turned to follow the pilot up to the cockpit, and he handed me

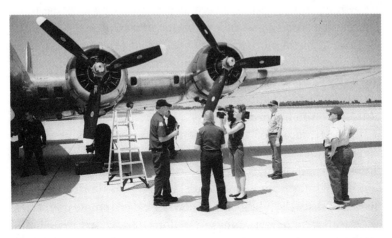

Interviewing a B-17 flight crew for a news story during my time at KHGI-TV in Nebraska.

a headset, then began the engine start-up procedure. The first engine roared to life, and the thunderous sound took my breath away. Soon, all four engines were running.

The pilot turned to me with a smile and a thumbs-up and started taxiing down the runway. Before long, we were airborne. My nerves settled as the plane reached altitude, but my mind stayed fixated on the plane's history. More than sixty years earlier, formations of B-17s had attacked Germany.

My view turned outward, to the bright sun shining down on the acres upon acres of green cornfields below. The sight was the perfect reminder that I was in the Cornhusker State, and it was my first moment of clarity that my new career was pretty special. Only a handful of airworthy B-17s were still in operation. Reporters are given access to some of the coolest experiences in life. Taking off in a Flying Fortress was one of my first.

"What do you think?" the pilot asked once we landed.

"I still can't believe I got to fly in a plane with so much history," I replied in a rush.

I relished my job that day and in the days to come.

The complexity of memory is significant in epilepsy and in the ways the disease impacts the brain and a person's quality of life. Everything from forming a sentence to following a recipe to remembering a vacation can be impacted by seizures.

Long-term memories are either implicit (unconscious) or explicit (conscious). Implicit memories include things like recalling lyrics to a song you haven't heard in five years and procedural memories like remembering how to ride a bike even if it's been ten years since you hopped on one.

Explicit memories include semantic—that is, your general knowledge of the world, such as the fact that the United States has fifty states and oranges are round—and episodic—like the lunch you had with a friend last month. Episodic memories from the distant past, like a childhood vacation, are called remote memories.

Within the context of these memories are verbal, visual, and spatial memories. For example, a verbal episodic memory is recalling a conversation with your best friend, while a visual episodic memory is recalling the setting where the conversation took place, like a coffee shop. A spatial memory is remembering where you parked the car when you left the coffee shop. Sometimes I would have a vague memory of a conversation with a friend but not the setting, or vice versa.

Then there is working memory. This allows someone to temporarily hold a limited amount of information to use immediately; if you're making cookies, for example, verbal working memory is following the steps to a recipe while no longer looking at the recipe, while visual-spatial working memory is remembering where you put the hot pad to get the cookies out of the oven. While reporting for KHGI-TV during that time, all my memory functions seemed to be operating just fine.

Outside of work, I was trying to carve out a social life. On one night out soon after moving to Nebraska, I met Nick, and he had me from hello. He was a few years older and lived in another town, so seeing each other around our work schedules wasn't easy. Nick was a banker, with normal working hours, and I was reporting on nights and weekends. One fall weekend, Christine and our friend Chris came into town, and Nick bought tickets to a Huskers football game for the four of us. A camera captured the laughter in our eyes as we posed for pictures from the stands, decked out in red Huskers T-shirts. We took more fun photos at a bar that night. Those pictures are the only proof I have of that day, because unlike the B-17 ride, I don't remember a single minute of it.

Unfortunately, our relationship was short-lived. My goal was to move on to a bigger TV market on one of the coasts in a couple of years. Nick's career and family were already planted in Nebraska. I tried to put thoughts of my career path on the backburner and just live in the moment because I really liked him, but it was clear that continuing a relationship with no future would just make things harder down the road. So we parted ways, and I promised myself I wouldn't date for the rest of my time in Nebraska.

Instead, I turned to my coworkers. The best part of working at a small station was that most of the other reporters and producers were also in their twenties. On days off we would often meet in

Kearney, a small college town where the TV station was located. Fun nights out for drinks and an awesome road trip to Colorado Springs to hike and to white-water raft one summer were captured in pictures. At the time I couldn't appreciate just how much I would come to value having those moments documented.

About a year into the job, I finally felt confident doing any type of story and decided I could handle a new challenge—a marathon.

After college, I had kept running, but took it easy. Training and competing had filled my schedule most of my life, so it was a relief to simply lace up my shoes and enjoy an eight-mile run without tracking my pace. But after a year away from it, the urge to compete returned. I missed training toward a goal. My longest race to this point was a 6K, but I was confident I could handle something longer. A 10K? Nah, I wasn't fast enough, and it didn't seem worthwhile to put in a lot of training to race that distance. How about a half marathon? Nah, why train so hard to run only half a race? If I was going to go in, I would go all in.

My younger brother Mike and I signed up for the 2008 Twin Cities Marathon, and I started training that summer, increasing my mileage from 30 to 45 a week. That's on the really low end for marathon training. Professionals run up to 120 miles per week, but I was an amateur and didn't want to risk getting hurt. Mike was also an amateur—a high school wrestler who wanted the challenge of a marathon, even though he didn't have time to train. I aimed for 7:10-minute miles, which would bring me in right under 3:10. I figured that was doable. The workouts were familiar, but where were the hills? Nebraska is flat, really flat. After a lot of running around, I managed to find inclines and pushed myself up and down them once a week.

In October, I drove back to Minneapolis, meeting my brother and our entire family for the event. Mike and I toed the start and took off at the gun. I settled into my race pace of 7:10 and warned myself to stay there. The biggest mistake distance runners make is going out too fast. I had trained hard enough to make my pace feel easy, at least until about mile 13. The athletes ahead were my motivation to push on, and I finished in 3:08, good enough to meet the Boston Marathon qualifying standard. My legs moved like bricks as I walked off the course, but I was elated. Since I made it out alive and healthy, I figured my body could handle another one. Racing had taken a backseat to reporting, and the marathon brought back my drive to push myself.

The May 2009 Lincoln National Guard Marathon in Nebraska was my next test. I followed the same training plan, but my legs were stronger this time and my heart was in better shape, so I had high expectations.

May 3 rolled around, and on a gorgeous, sunny morning in Lincoln, I joined a few hundred other anxious runners. We spaced out a bit to shake out our nerves, took a big breath, lined up at the starting line, and placed our index fingers on the start button of our watches. The gun went off along with dozens of beeps. I settled into a comfortable pace. My legs moved effortlessly along the flat course. A few miles into the race, I glanced to my right and then to my left. Men surrounded me. Up ahead, a few ponytails flying side to side pushed me to speed up. A marathon is a physical and mental race, full of inner dialogue about how to manage one's time.

It would be foolish to run faster to catch up at this point.

Don't lose sight of them. Just keep them in view.

And for the first fifteen miles or so, I did.

Then my stomach started cramping. Some people call it a side stitch. I called it "Oh shit. I have to stop."

And no, not at the porta potty. Thank God. The cramps hit in sharp jabs that forced me to stop because it was so hard to breathe. I stepped aside and stood frozen there for a minute, forcing myself to inhale slowly.

A few minutes of walking, a little water, and half a banana later, my stomach settled enough to start a slow jog. The cramps soon returned though, and so did my frustration.

Dammit, stupid stomach.

Stopping to walk again and again was the only choice I could make. The cycle of slow jog, cramps, and stop and walk continued seven times before my stomach finally settled down. I finally crossed the finish line in disappointment at 3:14. All my tough workouts had resulted in a worse time, not a better one.

As I was training for that marathon, my mom and Kara started to notice something was off. Kara noticed subtle lapses in my memory over the phone, like remembering details of a conversation we had had a month before. We both had been crisscrossing the country since college, and we usually caught up over the phone. In February 2009, I flew from Nebraska to Boston to see her and her fiancé, Ben. I don't remember that weekend, but Kara does.

"At times during your visit, you didn't act or seem at all like yourself," she recalled. "You were unpredictable. You would get angry easily, but then twenty minutes later, you were your old carefree self. I remember wanting to talk to you about it, but I was afraid. You definitely did not seem open to discussion."

Why did I get so upset so easily around my best friend? Especially on a vacation? That had never happened in high school or college, and I couldn't blame Keppra. This was four years later.

When it was time to head back to Nebraska, Kara dropped me off at the airport, bridesmaid dress in hand, and hugged me goodbye.

The dress didn't make it back. I forgot it at the airport.

To this day, I remember nothing from that trip to Boston. I figured any problems with memory were due to my fast-paced job and the need to take in and remember new things every day. So I pushed aside my forgetting the dress as a stupid mistake.

Just a few months after the marathon, the sun had not yet risen outside my studio apartment when I woke, a little dizzy, with a cramp in my neck. I rolled over and slowly gained focus to see the legs of a chair level with me.

I'm on the floor.

My body froze while my eyes darted around the room.

Where am I? Why am I on the floor?

I slowly propped myself up, recognizing the walls of my apartment after a minute. The sky outside my window was dark. My bed was tucked up beside the wall, and I was lying next to it on the rough, beige carpet.

I hadn't had any alcohol or a bad dream. So what had happened?

My mind quickly rewound to the seizures in my college apartment four years earlier. My fingers reached up to my face, gently touching my forehead, eyes, nose, and mouth.

No blood. No acute pain. No tender spots.

Whew.

But my gut filled with dread.

Was I on the floor because of a seizure?

I leaned against my bed with possible scenarios swimming through my head. Trying to make sense of something like this with zero clues was exasperating.

Do I need to see a doctor for this?

I didn't even understand what had happened, and I wasn't injured.

I stood up slowly and took a few tentative steps, then hesitantly walked toward the kitchen and back, my head swirling with what-ifs.

Eat breakfast and you'll feel better, I told myself.

A few hours later, I needed a mental break. The only way to calm my confused mind was to get moving. I changed clothes, tied up my shoes, and opened my apartment door. Then I stopped in my tracks.

Should I run? What if something weird happens again?

I turned and looked back at my bed, then the floor, then turned away. Sitting in my apartment, alone, stressing about the unknown would drive me crazy.

Take it easy, I thought, and if you feel weird and confused, STOP and come home.

I opened my door again and jogged down the steps into the crisp, cool air. The fresh air cleared my mind immediately, but not wanting to push my luck, I stopped after five miles. My body felt fine the entire time, and for the rest of the day, so I brushed the strange morning off. I didn't have any other incidents in the days and weeks to follow. Maybe it had been nothing more than a bad dream.

I shared the news with my mom. I didn't realize how much my parents worried about my health at that time. But while I had

largely forgotten about the seizures in college until this latest episode, my mom hadn't. Her instincts told her something was up.

"Somehow I either knew you were having seizures or sensed
that you were. Or maybe I was afraid you were. I really worried
about everything. One was a lack of sleep possibly triggering seizures. I worried about your running in the hot, hot, summer. I
worried about your driving back to Minnesota. I worried about you
going out with friends, knowing you wouldn't get enough sleep.
I didn't worry about your siblings like this. I didn't have to. So,
something was going on to cause me to worry so much," she later
told me.

For all the worrying my mom was doing about me, why wasn't
I worrying too?

5

Sleepless in Seattle

I loved my life in Nebraska, but it was time to move on to a new market. Most reporter contracts start out at two or three years, long enough to gain some great experience and to discover if you love the business enough to put up with the crazy hours and crappy pay. And I did. Showing up to work with no idea of what my day would look like made every day an adventure. As long as I got to shoot video, write, and edit my stories, I was happy. Now the choice was to stay in Nebraska or to go on another adventure.

I set my sights on the Pacific Northwest. The landscapes and active lifestyle inspired me to apply to a station in Eugene, Oregon, and I was thrilled when the KEZI 9 news director offered me the job. In December 2009, my mom helped me pack up my place, and we headed west.

The trip is ingrained in her memory, but not mine. I was at the wheel on a rural stretch of highway, singing along to the radio, when all of a sudden she felt the car slow down. My mom looked over at me in confusion, thinking something was wrong with the brakes. She recalls the look on my face.

"You were just staring into space. I had no idea this was a seizure, but I was scared. If we had been in heavy traffic, we would have been rear-ended. All of a sudden you came out of it and passed it off as nothing."

She took over the wheel. My brain gave me no clue that it had blacked out; it was like skipping past an exit sign without realizing it. I felt completely normal, and my mom's frantic tone seemed unnecessary. But then uneasiness started to creep in.

What song had I been singing along to? Blank. What had we been talking about? Blank. Why would I take my foot off the gas? Blank. None of it made sense.

Neither my friends nor my coworkers in Nebraska, including Steve, whom I saw the most, told me they ever noticed anything wrong. I chalked the experience up to fatigue from the last few days of working, packing, and saying my goodbyes. My brain must have simply shut down from exhaustion. But then I had a flashback to the strange incident in my apartment a few months before when I had woken up on the floor.

That time I fell. This time I basically zoned out, but I didn't crash the car or get injured. Both incidents were strange, but they only happened once. Don't dwell on it, I told myself.

Later that night at the motel, my mom witnessed another staring episode; this time I was brushing my hair at the sink.

"You brushed me off again when I asked you about it," she later told me.

Why would I stare into space and not notice it?

I decided to settle into my new apartment before determining whether I should see a neurologist. The problem seemed to have gone away on its own in college. Maybe it would again.

Driving into Eugene in December was like driving into one huge rain cloud. I peered out the passenger window at the bike and running paths as we navigated the college town, the windshield wipers on full throttle. This was my first time in the Pacific Northwest, and I was used to a mix of both gray and sun with Minnesota winters. The nearly constant cloudy winter skies of my new state would soon become a fitting analogy for my increasingly foggy memory.

The weather didn't bother me. Eugene is built for bikers and runners, with mulch trails winding for miles throughout the city. Referred to as TrackTown USA, it's the birthplace of Nike, a perfect place for pros, collegiate stars, and runners of all abilities to train. As soon as I saw the trails, I signed up for my next race, the 2010 Rock 'n' Roll Seattle Marathon.

My feet quickly covered many miles of the city, as I discovered beautiful new parks and paths. Some people seek out running groups in a new city, but as an introvert with an unusual work schedule, I found peace through simply jumping on a trail with my iPod and Garmin watch to push me along. I was excited to spend the next two years of my life here, taking in all that the region had to offer. Aside from traveling, I hoped to start dating again. But my reporting shift—2:30 p.m. to 11:30 p.m., including weekends— offered little opportunity for a personal life.

Walking into the TV station that first day was a little eye- opening, because I had never worked in a huge newsroom before, just a small bureau. Reporters' desks were grouped in pods of four, scattered throughout the spacious newsroom. The hustle and bus- tle took a little while to get used to, but I quickly began to love my new job. The new challenge here was finishing stories with earlier deadlines to leave time for a live shot. I loved the busy environment and accepted that it came with high pressure at times, fully aware that I might make a mistake. But the news must go on. If I had a bad day, I had to get over it, because a new day meant a new story.

Most of my coworkers were in their twenties, like me, and so our work and social lives began to overlap. The gorgeous coast and mountain ranges of Oregon, Washington, and northern California would become our road trip destinations. A few months into the job, my new friend and coworker Kate—a keenly perceptive and empathetic person, great qualities in a journalist and a friend— observed my confusion during conversations.

"You were spacey," she recalled. "You would forget important things in people's lives and ask about them again."

That's just how Christine described my junior year of college. I wished I could get inside my head in 2010. At what point did I start spacing out? How much did I miss?

Soon enough, other coworkers started to notice the blank look in my eyes during conversations. I couldn't recall a question I was asked or, more commonly, give the right answer. I'd look down and away in embarrassment, begging my brain to remember, but it was like trying to see through a dense fog.

Other times the lapse in awareness would take complete control of the conversation. These moments with coworkers started to get awkward. The signs were subtle but noticeable enough that they assumed I simply wasn't paying attention. I knew I seemed flighty but hoped it wasn't as bad as it seemed. Kate was honest with me, saying that I would completely zone out and stop talking midsentence. Disbelief filled each person's eyes. I tried to laugh off my confusion once I realized what had happened.

"Shoot, sorry, I got distracted. I'm kind of tired today."

But those moments would consume my thoughts for the rest of the night.

They must think I'm such a ditz.

Those fleeting moments were quickly forgotten because I was always on the go. For the first six months in Oregon, I focused hard on my training, sleep schedule, and work. The news was like sports—there was always room to improve—and without realizing it, I was applying an athlete's mindset to nearly everything that crossed my path.

But marathon training on top of a new job started catching up with me. The insomnia from college was working its way back into my life. My goal was eight hours of sleep a night, but I was waking up every hour, tossing and turning.

How can I think clearly at work if I'm numb from exhaustion?

Lying in bed, my attention would switch to the tough workouts ahead. The urge to look at the alarm clock, even though it would stress me out, was too strong to fight. I would roll over, straining to see the bright red numbers. 2:30 a.m. The digits glared back at me as if to say, "Good luck with your interval workout in a few hours; you can't half-ass your day and put a good story together if you're a zombie."

Coffee wasn't part of my life yet. My energy came solely from early morning workouts.

Was the sleep deprivation causing me to feel loopy and to randomly blank out?

Without a frame of reference, I assumed those weird moments were my brain trying to handle a mix of poor sleep, a new, fast-paced job, and hard physical training. I wasn't falling down and injuring myself, so things couldn't have been that serious, right?

I told myself I would go see a neurologist after the next marathon if things still felt weird.

Six months into my new job, it was time to race another 26.2 miles.

Nerves kept me up most of the night before the marathon, so with hardly three hours of poor sleep, I toed the starting line at 7:00 a.m. in Tukwila, Washington. The race would twist and turn along residential neighborhoods, lakes, and I-90 before ending at Qwest Field in downtown Seattle. The hill training I'd done didn't prepare me enough for the inclines that greeted me that morning. I was already exhausted, so the hills zapped most of my energy, and as any marathoner can attest, seeing flat land ahead was such a mental boost. Throbbing quads and hamstrings loosened up while my mind and body went back into autopilot. I sucked down an energy packet for one more jolt and glanced at the time.

2:51 . . . 2:52 . . .

My goal was 2:55, but I knew that as the race progressed, the hills would catch up to me, so I backed off.

Mile 24, check my watch.

Mile 25, check my watch.

The noise and music in the distance started getting louder, and the cheering crowd slowly came into view. I felt the support as I glanced down at my watch and pushed toward the finish. The large race clock above the finish came into view, and I wiped the sweat dripping off my forehead and squinted into the sun to see 2:59, with the seconds ticking away. I'd been pounding my feet into concrete for almost three hours, but nothing was more important to me than the next thirty seconds. They would determine if all my training and sleepless nights had been worth it.

On this day, I willed myself to the finish line, looking up to see the clock at 2:59:56 with music thumping. A photo captured my tired smile but also the twinkle in my eye. It's the look of accomplishment any athlete understands, knowing that all their training had paid off.

My true time was 2:59:48. Breaking three hours was decided in just eleven seconds. I came in third place running on just three hours of sleep. My hands dropped to my knees as I bent forward

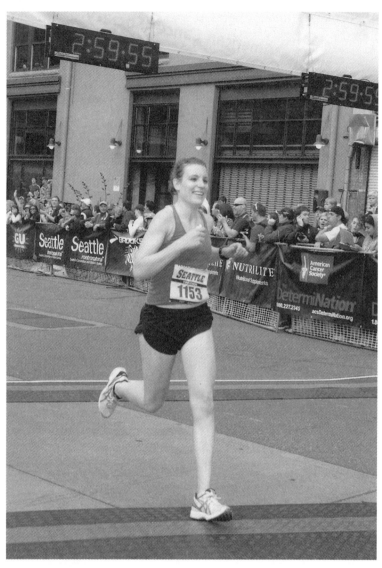

Crossing the finish line during the Rock 'n' Roll Seattle Marathon.

in exhaustion, but my brain was too high on endorphins to notice any pain. A race organizer approached and handed over a huge, shiny framed third-place certificate. To my surprise, I also won a $1,000 check.

I shuffled toward a water station with the award under my arms, nodding at other competitors with a weak smile. After some small talk, I jogged away from the music to make an excited call to my mom, dad, and Kara.

I had set a goal and achieved it without getting injured. It was the first time I had truly been proud of my performance since running a 3,000-meter race in college, when I achieved a new personal record by fifteen seconds. In that moment it struck me how a few seconds can mean the difference between pure joy and utter frustration.

After picking up my gear bag, I headed for the nearby pier for lunch and then to the Pike Place Fish Market to pick up some smoked salmon. I stepped out into the warm June sun for a stroll around the busy pier to loosen up my aching body. Seagulls flew in and perched next to me on a fence. The picture-perfect view brought a big smile to my face before the drive home to Eugene.

I dragged my feet into my apartment around five o'clock that afternoon, wanting nothing more than a long hot shower and a satisfying dinner. The marathon endorphins had worn off as exhaustion set in.

Doctors tell people who experience seizures to avoid risky activities like swimming and rock climbing. Preparing any food that requires a sharp knife should be added to the list of cautions. Carrots lay in front of me, and I started to chop. Without any indication of a seizure or of how much time had passed, I came to and looked around in a daze, soon realizing the cold kitchen floor was beneath me.

"Where am I?" I called out nervously.

But there was no one to answer me. My head slowly circled to see a fridge, a dishwasher—and then blood on the floor. Panic hit as I quickly followed the path of blood up my body, then spotted the streaks all over my left arm. I turned my wrist and jolted back in shock to see blood still slowly trickling out of the long incision.

"Shit!! What is this?" I took in a quick, short breath.

I gripped my arm to put pressure over the cut until the bleeding stopped, exhaling slowly, scanning the floor for clues.

Less than a foot away lay the small paring knife. My pulse quickened as I reached for it, then turned away in disgust at the sight. I pulled myself up onto my knees and reached for it again, knowing how dangerous it would be for the knife to remain in the middle of the floor. Sticky blood covered the handle and my hands.

"Ugh, gross," I groaned.

Gross, yes, but at least the handle was easy to grip. With knife in hand, I grabbed the counter with my other hand to pull myself up. A wave of dizziness hit me, nearly knocking me back down. The knife dropped into the sink. I leaned over the counter until the lightheadedness passed, then blasted cold water and soap over my arm to wash off the remaining streaks of red. After wiping the cut dry with a paper towel, I looked it over. The red incision on my arm was a good six inches long. The knife in the sink gleamed in the light. Without picking it up, I played out in my head what must have happened. The seizure must have struck as I was slicing into the carrot, with the knife slipping down to slice through my forearm instead.

I stared down at the incision, realizing in that moment how close it was to a major artery, the ulnar artery.

"Seriously? Did this really just happen?" I whispered.

I rummaged through my cupboard to find Band-Aids. Disbelief washed over me as I placed five adhesive strips horizontally over the cut. I was exasperated—a seizure had put a quick end to what had been a really great day.

Why had the seizures from college come back? It had been five years since my last one.

That question would take ten years to answer.

Now for the knife. My hands shook slightly as I picked it up, forcing me to look down at the sharp blade to avoid cutting myself again. After a quick scrub and rinse, I stuck it on the drying rack next to the sink and grabbed paper towels to wipe up the floor. But a glance up at the knife as I bent down gave me chills and made me stop. The clean silver sparkled, as though nothing had happened.

Hiding this scar would be impossible in the spring and summer.

With a big sigh, I stood up, carefully placed the knife into a drawer and turned to leave the kitchen. But a few steps later an image of the blade reappeared. Out of sight wasn't enough; out of mind was only possible if that thing was in the garbage, never to meet my skin again. Heck, the thought of anything sharp in my apartment now felt unsettling. My knives were relatively new and expensive, but I didn't care. I picked up the entire set, walked over to the garbage can, and almost dropped it in before spotting the plastic bag. Logic screamed out.

"You can't do that!! Those will puncture the bag!"

Defeated, I set the knife back on the counter and stared at it for a few seconds. The only place for it to go now was in my car. I don't remember where I brought the set the next day. This was definitely not something my parents needed to find out about. A seizure was one thing. Slicing an arm open during a seizure was another. Roughly nine hours earlier, we had all been in good spirits, and this would ruin their day nearly as much as it had ruined mine.

My mom wouldn't find out until a few years later, when she helped unpack boxes at my new apartment and noticed the knives were missing. She never asked about them. An expensive set of new knives had disappeared. Intuition told her something had happened. She later told me that she figured I either gave the set away or threw it out.

That night, I finally wiped up the floor, ate a huge bowl of cereal, brushed my teeth, took a shower, and fell into bed, too exhausted to see straight anymore. Going to the emergency room never crossed my mind. Aside from the cut on my arm I hadn't seriously hurt myself, so why max out my insurance deductible?

I woke up Sunday morning after a solid twelve hours of sleep, but it wouldn't be enough to calm the neurons short-circuiting across my brain. At some point I confided to Kate what had happened. The details escaped me when I started writing this book;

she reminded me that seizures had struck all weekend long. I didn't know at the time that repeated seizures could be deadly—I wasn't on medication to stop the firestorms in my brain.

Nothing could disguise the cuts and bruises on my face Monday morning. I'm not a person to call in sick for anything, so on went the makeup with extra concealer, and out the door I went. My efforts to hide my black eye were unsuccessful. Kate noticed. So did everyone else.

The knife and the blood scared me. Waking up in a pool of blood is what it took for me to finally talk to a neurologist. I could no longer deny that something wasn't right.

6

Calming the Storm

After a round of phone calls on Monday, I got lucky. A neurologist at PeaceHealth Medical Group had an opening for an appointment in two days. I felt apprehensive but optimistic when I walked into the RiverBend Pavilion in Springfield, Oregon. Five years had passed since my last neurology appointment in Minneapolis, but with all the moving around to new jobs, the clock seemed to have ticked at warp speed.

After a short wait, a nurse ushered me into an examination room. Dr. James Kiley walked in a few minutes later. Tall and lanky, he greeted me with a handshake and a friendly hello.

I explained about the incident with the knife, my disorientation following the marathon in Seattle, and the strange zoning out at work. Then he said the word I had turned a deaf ear and a blind eye to for months, the word I had refused to connect my symptoms with and had avoided seeing a doctor for, in fear of the diagnosis. Dr. Kiley typed his diagnosis into my medical notes.

"It sounds like she has temporal lobe epilepsy, and occasionally has secondary generalizations."

A surge of excessive electrical activity in one part of the brain—like the temporal or frontal lobe—is called a focal seizure because the seizure has a focus. If the seizure spreads and jumps to the other hemisphere, that's called a secondary generalized seizure. Seizures that begin in both hemispheres of the brain at once are called generalized seizures. Tonic-clonics are an example.

A few things must happen for a seizure to develop. First is location: the seizure focus provides the physiological spark to start the seizure. Next, an initiating circuit, which is a separate group of neurons outside the focus area, is needed to convert the spark into a seizure. Some seizures start and end in the same area. But for a seizure to spread, it must recruit nearby regions of the brain. Once the routes are laid down, seizures will take them again and again, sometimes to a neighboring lobe, sometimes to the other hemisphere. All this time, seizures are being regulated by modulatory centers, which affect the seizure's intensity, its duration, and the likelihood it will spread. The brain's chemistry actually changes during a seizure, which causes it to spread.

Seizures develop differently for everyone, and epilepsy can be hard to diagnose based on symptoms alone. My episodes of zoning out looked like absence seizures, a type of generalized epilepsy where people will stare off into space for three to twenty seconds, then return to normal right away. It's like turning off the lights and turning them right back on. Absence seizures can happen multiple times a day.

The other type—which Dr. Kiley thought I had—is called focal impaired awareness seizures. They start in one part of the brain, usually alter awareness for thirty seconds or longer, and can cause confusion afterward. This matched my experience; I would regain awareness but have no clue what I missed.

At first the seizures seemed to stay isolated to zoning out. But after the weekend following the marathon in Seattle, my brain never really returned to normal. Seizures started spreading and sometimes grew into tonic-clonics.

I needed to start medication as soon as possible because the seizures were turning into firestorms. The source of those fires wasn't being controlled, so the flames were pushing across the landscape of my brain, forcing me to the ground in convulsions and leaving injuries in their wake.

Antiseizure medications (ASMs) work by either altering electrical activity in neurons or altering chemical transmission between neurons. Dozens of ASMs are on the market, but no two brains are the same, and there's no guarantee the first, second, or third drug will successfully control seizures.

Dr. Kiley prescribed a new drug called Vimpat and gave me some samples. Relief washed over me when I gazed down at the tiny pills. I thanked him and left the clinic, happy and hopeful. But he made it clear that ASMs often only work alongside the same lifestyle rules I had tried to follow since college: good sleep, exercise, healthy food, and no or little alcohol. A seven- or eight-hour night of sleep is a luxury for some adults; for me, it was potentially lifesaving. Neurons in my brain functioned normally when I was rested, but dipping below seven hours of sleep a night was like waking a sleeping giant.

Could the ASMs control what was triggering my firestorms?

I wouldn't get enough time to find out.

Those little pills cost a lot, more than $1,000 a month. My health insurance wouldn't cover the cost, and a generic option wasn't available, so Dr. Kiley started me on another medication, Lamotrigine. My hopes were high that it would work.

As a journalist, the most logical thing I could do was to start researching my diagnosis, but I did so tentatively. Curiosity and fear played tug-of-war in my head; I didn't want to find all my symptoms online and trust Dr. Google to predict my future. So my fingers stayed away from the search engine at first.

The cut on my arm and other dangerous falls stayed in the back of my mind though, and it soon became obvious that living alone was not smart. Moving in with two roommates ended up being one of the best things I could do for my health. The house was in a nice neighborhood near the Amazon Trail, a figure-eight-shaped running path covered by a canopy of trees in some areas and flanked by wide-open grassland in others. You could always bump into someone training for a race—the mile-long route was perfect for intervals, and it connected to another, longer trail. The soft, wood-chip surface and calming scenery became my favorite place for workouts.

Luckily, a great bike path lined the street outside my new neighborhood too. Dr. Kiley took my driving privileges away, in compliance with Oregon law, which requires one to be seizure free for a certain time period before driving. Now my only option to get to work, rain or shine, was on two wheels.

A week into the new medication, I was seizure free and happy to share the news with my parents. My mom was hard at work researching epilepsy and emailed me with an update:

"Stacia, my mind can't get off of the fact of how great you're feeling with your medication. I'm so happy for you. When I was watching your stories last night, it was so good to know you did those while feeling good and not having to worry about the next seizure. I'm on my way over to the library to pick up the magazine on seizures, so keep your fingers crossed it's in!"

A smile spread across my face. Seeing my mom happy brought me relief. I wanted the seizures gone as much for my parents as for me—when they worried, I worried. The note of confidence in her email gave me more faith that the medicine could truly work. I got a taste of success—one week of work without black eyes and bruises or confusion of my surroundings—and I didn't want that feeling to vanish.

The drug is working! I feel great, so it's fine to drive a little bit, just a short trip, just to get some groceries.

I made it there and back without a hitch.

My confidence rose higher. Could taking a few ASMs a day really end the seizures? Would my luck last?

It didn't take long for the answer: an unequivocal "NO."

Kate recalls the night I returned to the TV station with one of our photojournalists, Heather, following a live shot. I fell into a wall hard enough that a chunk of drywall broke off. The seizure left behind its mark once again with abrasions to my face.

For a career that required driving and appearing on camera, this was beyond exasperating. KEZI graciously accommodated me by changing my work schedule so I could work with Heather. She drove us to stories, and though I was grateful to keep reporting, losing my independence was tough on both of us. It wasn't Heather's job to be my chauffeur. She was a very talented photojournalist, and it led to some tense moments between us. We wanted to shoot, write, and edit our own stories.

Buckling up in the passenger's seat made me feel like a burden. At that point, I had never considered epilepsy to be a disability, partly because I was under the impression that epilepsy was a brain disorder, not a disease. "Brain disorder" didn't sound as serious. The International League Against Epilepsy changed the definition of epilepsy from "disorder of the brain" to "disease of the brain" in 2014, saying that "disorder" implies epilepsy is a temporary disturbance of the brain and so minimizes its seriousness. Epilepsy is a chronic disease that causes repeated seizures.

Epilepsy is covered under the Americans with Disabilities Act, but I felt as if the word "disability" didn't apply to me because the seizures didn't seem bad enough. I understood that word to be reserved for people who couldn't hold down a job because their epilepsy was so debilitating. Not being able to drive was my biggest issue; it was hard to see everyone else simply grab a set of keys and hustle out the door to their interviews. Sometimes I told myself, "Be grateful you have a driver and don't dwell on what other people think of your seizures." But standing on the sidelines in a competitive work environment was upsetting.

Dr. Kiley increased my medication, which gave me hope again. At first glance, the statistics looked promising. ASMs control seizures for approximately two-thirds of adults with epilepsy in the United States, meaning most people live seizure free. Some people do for years, or for decades, or even for the rest of their lives.

But if Lamotrigine failed to control my seizures, I only had a good shot at one more ASM. Doctors sometimes pair two or three ASMs together, hoping to find the perfect combination. But extensive research shows that if two drugs fail to completely control seizures, it's unlikely a third one will. Thankfully, those stats weren't relayed to me. An epilepsy diagnosis was tough enough. I would have fallen apart if someone added, "Oh, and your type of seizures is the hardest to treat. Brain surgery might be your only chance."

Bad news needs to be spaced out, one piece at a time, otherwise there's no room for hope to squeeze in. Hope is what I held onto.

Running had been holding me together, but it was getting riskier. Every step I took could bring me closer to another seizure.

Heather became witness to precisely how often my brain was short-circuiting. She and Kate estimated I'd had hundreds of seizures that year. I later discovered that some of those moments of disorientation were not in fact seizures but something called the postictal state.

The postictal state is the altered state of consciousness following a seizure as the brain recovers and returns to baseline. Symptoms during the postictal state can range from confusion and memory loss to mood disorders, aggression, and more. Like gray thunderclouds sprinkling down the last droplets of rain before the sun appears again, the brain too slowly wakes up from a brutal brainstorm, in a state of confusion that can last anywhere from a few seconds to a few days. At that time, my postictal state typically lasted five to thirty minutes, sometimes longer. My confusion mimicked some of my seizure symptoms. Regardless of what state of mind I was in, it wasn't the best for working in live TV. One night, a seizure forced Heather to call the station and cancel my live shot.

Missing that live shot was a low point for me. Having seizures at work was one thing, but putting producers in a bind to fill thirty seconds in a newscast because I suddenly couldn't go live was another.

I hated epilepsy in those moments. It held the reins. I was powerless.

You're a burden, Stacia. Don't be a burden.

The word started filtering into my thoughts more and more as my independence evaporated. I thought things couldn't get much worse, but one night in 2010 I had a seizure on-air at the end of an interview with the mayor of Eugene. Kate witnessed it.

"The mayor thought things had wrapped up," Kate recalled. "She thought she was done with the interview, and then you turned and stared straight into the lens of the camera and didn't say anything."

The production crew immediately cut back to the anchors, and I went back to the station upset with myself. I had hoped that day would never come, but now the embarrassment forced me to sit down and think about what was truly provoking these seizures. Seizures didn't always strike after a bad night of sleep. So, let's see, stress? Poor sleep stressed me out, but it wasn't stress alone, because then they'd be happening every day around deadline at work.

What else did I do consistently? I ran.

No article I'd read noted running as a trigger, and I didn't exercise every day, but when I did . . .

I stood up from the couch, walked over to my desk, picked up my phone, and tapped on the calendar.

Oh shoot, what days did I take off?

Racking my brain, I stared at the calendar, hoping a few days would pop out. Today was Friday.

Did I run last Friday? I don't think so, but Saturday, yes. And there was a seizure Saturday night. I slept a lot that night, so Sunday's run was OK. Did I run Monday? No clue. Tuesday? Probably. Wednesday? Yes. Thursday? Yes.

The schedule was pretty similar each week, so I added up more dates.

The weekend seizures I could remember, and those happened on days I ran. But what about other seizures? I sighed. This is why doctors want patients to keep a seizure journal. But I didn't. I was convinced seizures would stay dormant if I kept my sleep consistent. Although I might have forgotten a day or two, I started putting two and two together. Running after a good night's rest went great. But after a night or two of tossing and turning, a seizure would send me into la-la land while running on my favorite trail.

At first, the seizures occurring after less than six and a half to seven hours of sleep seemed to happen sporadically, but now they were happening consistently. Sleep was gas in the tank, I realized. Not enough left me sputtering to a stop on the road, hoping someone could come by to guide me home. At work, sleep was gas in the tank to get through interviews and live shots without breaking down.

Now that the pieces of the puzzle fit, it was obvious that running while tired was like walking on eggshells. The one thing sending my exhausted brain over the edge was completely in my control 100 percent of the time. No one was forcing me to tie my shoes and push my body out the door.

7

Déjà Vu

"You and I were side by side on the elliptical."

My sister remembers the day well. We were home for the holidays in December 2011. I had flown to Colorado and caught a ride with Kara and Ben to Thief River Falls. The day after Christmas, antsy to get out of the house, Sara and I headed to the gym to work off our Christmas cookies. Peanut butter blossoms were our weakness, and mom made too many. The fourteen-hour drive home put a dent in my sleep schedule, so I decided to stay off the treadmill and chose the elliptical machine instead.

Maybe I'll be less likely to have a seizure if I'm not running.

Sara jumped on the elliptical right next to me. We matched stride for stride for the first twenty minutes or so. But in her peripheral vision she noticed me slow down, so she turned to see me staring straight ahead with a blank expression. She jumped off her machine.

"I suddenly got scared. I knew you had seizures, but I had never seen one. I said your name a few times and touched your arm, not sure what to do. You snapped out of your daze and looked around and asked where you were," she recollected.

Sara stood nervously next to me. Ben happened to be at the gym and saw my confusion. They both gently tried to convince me to go home, but once I realized I was on an elliptical and a seizure had interrupted my workout, Sara said, I started moving my legs again and told them I wanted to stay for another thirty minutes.

"I didn't know what to do, or what was best for you at that point," she recalled. "I wanted your life to go on as normal as much as you did."

Back to normal. There's nothing I wanted more. So why did I dismiss Sara's and Kate's concerns? "Normal" to me meant holding down a job and working out like everyone else. I stayed too busy to become fearful. But now I can see that brushing Sara and Kate off put the fear on their shoulders, something I regret.

And so the cycle continued—sleep well, miss one night of good sleep, have a seizure, sleep for twelve hours to recover, and wake up ready to go again. I was becoming less afraid, fearless in a way.

Fearlessness is taking a risk, realizing that you might fail or that something bad could happen. And even if it does, you pick yourself up and try to do it differently next time. The concept worked to my advantage at first. I wasn't afraid of getting lost when I went running. My attitude carried over to my job. A career in television journalism requires its own level of fearlessness. News reporters enter their stations most days unaware of what the day could bring. We usually interview strangers, stopping them outside to ask their views on a range of issues, knocking on their doors to ask about a death in the family or in the neighborhood. We're aware the door might slam in our faces, we may forget our lines during a live shot, or we may get a cruel letter from a viewer. And on some occasions we could agree to a high-risk assignment. Being fearless can sometimes bring success, but with epilepsy, you need to recognize your limits.

I didn't let myself chance it anymore on little sleep, but if I slept well, I headed out the door. Striking the crunchy mulch, stride after stride, gave me energy and cleared my mind.

After the wave of seizures following the Rock 'n' Roll Seattle Marathon in June 2010, I knew I shouldn't train for another marathon. The scar on my arm is a daily reminder of how awful that weekend had been. I decided to run just for fun and only when my body was rested.

So that's what I did at first. The wet, foggy winter mornings often left me with soggy shoes but also a smile on my face. Being healthy enough to exercise was a gift. The runner's high is real, and coming home out of breath was like lifting a weight off my shoulders.

But the fun became too easy—my legs craved the burning sense of accomplishment that only came from a hard workout. Running at an easy pace on the same trails I used to train on didn't help.

While I ran, images of competition started to resurface.

You're already on the trail. Just pick up the pace.

So I did, and I was surprised by how fit I still was seven months after the marathon. As those winter months passed and my feet picked up speed, some vivid details of how truly scary that night after Seattle had been started to fade, along with the scar on my arm. The faster I got, the harder it was to turn off my Garmin. My internal struggle was in moving forward, not backing off.

You can run faster. You know you can. Just get more sleep this time.

One thing runners are good at—runners I know, anyway—is asking why the last race hadn't gone so great and figuring out what we could do differently to achieve a new personal record the next time. It's part of competing; there's always room for improvement because your performance is tied to a stopwatch. The more you race, the more you understand your body and how hard you can push it.

Subconsciously, I was using a similar mindset in managing epilepsy.

Each seizure taught me how far I could push myself, how much sleep deprivation I could get away with before my brain rebelled.

I told myself this: I had not been prepared enough for Seattle's hills, and I beat up my tired body for 26.2 miles. My brain responded with multiple seizures. There's my explanation. What could I do differently next time? Train harder on hills and get more sleep before the race. Boom. Problem solved. I knew I could drop ten minutes. It wasn't an easy goal, but it wasn't unattainable either. So, I signed up for the Eugene Marathon and started training that winter for the May 2011 race.

Someone could logically ask, "Why wouldn't you just stop running if it triggered seizures? Couldn't you go for bike rides instead?"

Biking was for my commute, and I didn't want to start over in a new sport. Buying a nice bike and training new muscles didn't appeal to me because I knew there was no guarantee I'd be any good at racing.

The train harder/sleep more plan for the Eugene Marathon worked, at first.

Then lights started flickering. A new type of storm was moving in.

The flicker was so quick. A split second of light . . . and my head instinctively turned to the ceiling to study the overhead light.

Was the bulb burning out?

Without blinking, I stared for three or four seconds and . . . nothing.

Weird. It had definitely flickered.

I shrugged my shoulders and sat down at the kitchen table. Immediately, a weird, uneasy feeling washed over me. My body froze; my breathing halted.

Something's not right.

Then, out of the corner of my eye, another flash of bright light.

Ok, the bulb must be going out . . . but . . .

It wasn't. It was exactly the opposite.

An electrical storm had already started rolling in, and the flashes of light were warnings that a larger seizure was on the way. I froze in fear.

I didn't know at the time that the warnings had a name—auras. They are the first symptom of a focal aware seizure, but not everyone gets them.

I stayed aware of my surroundings, but disturbing sensations like flickering lights crept in, and it wouldn't take long for other strange feelings to appear. Auras were unsettling because I was conscious but knew things weren't right. Not until I started to learn more about seizures did I realize that auras can arrive as swirling colors, vivid memories, tastes, smells, rising nausea, a sense of impending doom, and more.

As unsettling as they were, and were about to get, I was grateful for the warning. Auras are a ticking clock to find a safe, private place before the seizure spreads and impacts awareness, becoming a focal impaired awareness seizure. Different seizures alter consciousness in different ways, depending on where in the brain the seizure starts and spreads. Some people may look awake and stay upright, but they aren't aware of their surroundings. That was me running on the trails in Eugene. A change in a person's behavior is the big clue—laughing, staring, crying, screaming, lip smacking, wandering around, or odd body posturing are signs of focal impaired awareness seizures.

At this point, the flickering lights, the staring into space, and the tonic-clonics were not completely controlled by medication. I didn't fully see my seizures as serious enough yet, though, only later realizing that the words "seizure" and "serious," with only a few letters separating the two, are similar for a reason.

The auras yet to come—déjà vu and jamais vu—forced me to confront how scary it was to get lost inside my own head. Once details of larger seizures came to light, I took the warnings even more seriously. Seizures can become more severe if they aren't controlled.

////

The gray sweater caught my eye first. Every night I picked out an outfit for work the next day, so that evening I opened my closet door, flipped on the light switch, and walked over to the long row of blouses, sweaters, and dresses. Just as I reached up for the sweater on its hanger, everything suddenly, but slowly, became still. Time slowed to the pace of a falling feather while my heart rate sped up and my breathing turned shallow. The world around me slowly faded away into the shadows. My finger lightly grazed the soft fabric, but my sense of touch had disappeared. I gulped, then carefully examined the tops in front of me, trying hard to make sense of their design and color. The fluorescent light above cast a familiar glow over the red and purple blouses.

Why does this look familiar?

Dread rose in my stomach as a growing uneasiness sank in— and kept sinking.

You already walked in here and picked out a gray top for tomorrow, right?

I turned my back to my clothes in hopes it would pass, but I knew this feeling well, and it frightened me.

Black flats next to the closet captured my attention next. I studied them intently for a few seconds. They hadn't moved. The shimmer of my silver Tiffany's necklace across the bedroom caught my gaze next.

That's the same necklace you picked up earlier, right?

A familiar but unsettling reality then washed over me.

This was not real.

I was experiencing déjà vu, meaning "already seen." It's an overwhelming, disturbing sense that I'd already lived this exact same moment before, that I had already walked into my bedroom and picked out that sweater and those shoes tonight.

But I hadn't.

Even the ambience of the bedroom and the light peeking in from the hallway were familiar, as if I was walking back onto a movie set. My brain was tricking me, but this was no joke. Maybe you've experienced déjà vu, a strong, intense feeling that you've done something identical before. I had experienced it before I developed epilepsy. But I can tell you that epileptic déjà vu is much more intense.

Déjà vu is a false feeling of familiarity. The illusion is believed to involve the areas of the temporal lobe that control our memory and emotions.

The hippocampus processes memory and the amygdala processes emotion. We have two of each. They are located in both the right and the left temporal lobes, just above the ears, and they work together to record and consolidate memories so they can be transferred to the cortex for long-term storage.

Seizures can start anywhere in a person's right or left temporal lobe. There is not clear evidence that repeated seizures cause progressive, permanent damage in the hippocampus, except for status epilepticus, which is an episode of repetitive prolonged seizures lasting more than five minutes. Seizures do cause circuits in the brain to change in other ways.

My current epileptologist, Dr. Jessica Winslow at the Minnesota Epilepsy Group, says that even if the hippocampus does not appear abnormal on imaging there can still be dysfunction with changes in its signaling and connections, and it could be a critical pathway for the seizure to spread. These issues can cause severe problems with a person's ability to form memories.

Sometimes—on a lucky day—my déjà vu faded into reality and the seizure stopped there, leaving me bewildered and tired. But soon enough, like the flickering lights, it became a warning sign that a larger seizure was on the way. As disturbing as déjà vu was, it wasn't as scary as jamais vu, which would also soon become a warning sign. Jamais vu is the exact opposite—the term means "never seen." Within about five seconds, a familiar area turns unfamiliar, like walking into your kitchen and having no clue where you are.

Nothing would scare me as much as that seizure I experienced along the Amazon Trail about one month before the 2011 Eugene Marathon. Familiarity was comforting during hard workouts, so this trail and the overcast skies should have made for a perfect day. No sun was beating down my back or blinding my vision. But on that spring morning, the clouds above couldn't guide my way once jamais vu crept in. I knew I was in the midst of a seizure while running but was powerless to stop it. My arms were pumping but my hands were tied. I slowed down and lost all awareness at some point.

When I regained awareness on the wet mulch, life would not carry on as usual right away. My brain transitioned into the postictal state, leaving me confused and disorientated and asking questions even if I was the only one around.

"Where am I?"

Now I was fully aware that things weren't right, and it was unsettling not to have answers.

"Where am I? What day is it?"

Emotions soon bubbled to the surface, and thankfully the couple who found me disoriented that spring day guided me home. The voices of those two caring strangers helped me finally see the reality I had been running from, and that was the first time I really broke down, angry that seizures were now completely overtaking the two things I loved—reporting and running. For the last ten months since the marathon in Seattle, I'd done my best to sleep enough but never made it to 100 percent.

Anyone who seeks out challenges in life understands the risk is for the reward, and I had been too driven and stubborn to realize the reward wasn't worth the risk in the long run.

Was it worth compromising my health solely for a 2:50 marathon time? Would dropping nine minutes from my Seattle time really matter in the big picture?

I knew I didn't need to race. Racing wasn't my career, nor is it for most people. Yet, we train to see all our hard work—thirteen- to twenty-four-mile Sunday runs, 800-meter and 1,600-meter intervals, tempo runs, grueling hill workouts, and strength training—pay off to line up for just one 5K, 10K, half marathon, or full marathon. Chasing a faster time becomes addicting. Tough workouts and races in college against some extremely talented teammates taught me how to push harder. But not anymore. My brain was pushing back. And my rationalizations for training were no longer valid. I realized that medication alone would never stop the firestorms. Marathon training was over.

A few days later, I laced up my shoes for a short run and felt a tug at my heel. My right Achilles tendon suddenly flared up.

Dammit!

If I needed a sign that marathon training was truly over, there it was.

Dr. Kiley had been on top of my seizures since day one. After my first appointment in June 2010, his nurse called me every month for the first six months to check how often I was having seizures. Dr. Kiley checked my blood levels each time and upped my meds. I accepted early on that it might take a while to get to a therapeutic dose strong enough to prevent a seizure. I told myself to be patient. But it was getting hard to take my own advice.

Seizures came and went in spurts; right when my dose went up a bit, they stopped, and I would let myself believe once again that I had finally found the magic dose. But the brainstorms always found new ways to break through the barrier of medication. My primary care doctor prescribed Ambien and recommended I see a sleep specialist, but I didn't want to take off any time from work nor pay to see more specialists. I was young. Sleep didn't seem like something I should have to pay a ton of money to figure out. I expected the Ambien to help at least somewhat. But it didn't, and my seizures only got worse.

Eight months of tweaking doses had yet to completely pay off. Lowering my marathon time and improving my skills as a reporter had been big personal goals. Both were races against the clock. I couldn't yet know whether an end to training would improve my outcome with epilepsy, but I did have a mindset switch. My belief that I was young and healthy enough to live a normal life, work crazy hours, run even crazier hours, and maintain a fun social life finally faded.

My social life still existed with coworkers, but my dating life was nonexistent. At twenty-five, I took my social cues from women on *The Bachelor*, who at my age fretted in dramatic fashion that their lives would be over if they didn't get engaged soon. The mid-twenties mantra to "get married and start having kids" echoes loudly for many Midwesterners. Thankfully, I was surrounded by women who were career focused at that time, so we held *Bachelor* watch parties and predicted the winners.

I couldn't fight my own reality. Dating took a back seat to sleep. Most of my weekends were spent in darkness, by way of either a seizure or attempts to sleep, which doesn't exactly work in the dating world. The thought of having an aura, much less a larger seizure, around a guy I barely knew made me hesitant. Explaining an aura over drinks. Now, there's a great conversation starter.

I wanted to date, but not at the expense of suffering more blackouts at work. Every incident made me less reliable and more self-conscious. The seizure that struck during a live shot with Eugene's mayor crushed my confidence, but it also reinforced the need to focus hard on each assignment.

Any story could be my last if a seizure seriously injured me.

The thought was both unbelievable and too real, and I often brushed it aside—nothing had come close enough yet.

But at least seizures won't kill me or cause any serious problems like some chronic diseases can, I told myself.

Unfortunately, I was very wrong.

8

A Difficult Patient

Everyone with epilepsy lives with the chance they won't wake up after their next seizure. The risk of premature death in people with epilepsy is up to three times higher than for the general population, according to the World Health Organization. Unlike many neurological diseases that can lead to death progressively (ALS, Alzheimer's disease, brain cancer), epilepsy is a chronic disease that people can live with for decades, but it can also kill within minutes. Sudden Unexplained Death in Epilepsy occurs when someone with epilepsy dies unexpectedly, usually in their sleep. Possible causes include disruptions with breathing functions and heart rhythm, both known to happen during seizures. People with uncontrollable seizures have a higher risk. Status epilepticus can also cause death. Tragically, suicide is another deadly consequence of the disease, as are seizure-related aspiration pneumonia and accidents.

Seizures can leave a person vulnerable like nothing else, without any control over where they are the moment one strikes. It's like being in the worst place at the worst time: boiling water on the stove or pulling food out of a hot oven, walking up or down a staircase, swimming in a pool or taking a bath, riding a bike or downhill skiing, and more. Normal things people do every day. If the paring knife that sliced my inner forearm while cutting vegetables had made contact one inch to the left, it would have hit my ulnar artery. A large bleed needs to be stopped immediately, not five minutes after coming out of a seizure. Falls are some of the most common accidents. My roommate said he caught me once during a seizure before I hit the floor. He timed each tonic-clonic, knowing that if one lasted more than five minutes he would need to call an ambulance.

I had put the thought of another accident on the back burner when my unpredictable mood took center stage. Why was I getting so upset and emotional at the drop of a hat so randomly? Aside from some sibling fights and thrown tennis rackets, in the past any irritation had always been directed inward. I hated drama and tried hard to avoid it with friends or coworkers. I was self-critical, a perfectionist on the track and in the studio, but also carefree in other aspects of life, as Kara reminded me. So there was a balance.

Now I was off-balance. My mood turned into a roller coaster; the ups and downs felt uncontrollable, wreaking havoc on both my personal and my professional life. I could go for hours in a good mood but then something small would flip my day upside down. Spats started occurring with coworkers, people I got along with fine when I started. Now I was a hot mess.

Was this due to the epilepsy itself? The stress of seizures? My medication?

Turns out, it could have been all of the above.

In temporal lobe epilepsy, my diagnosis from Dr. Kiley, the amygdala can generate too much emotion. It's just one part of the limbic system, which controls mood and exchanges signals with the rest of the brain. Research shows that depression is common in people with temporal lobe epilepsy. My problem wasn't depression; it was moodiness. The bursts of anger seemed so random at times, and I think fatigue played into some of it. Fatigue also made me more prone to seizures.

I described the symptoms I experienced in Oregon to Dr. Edward Bertram, professor of neurology at the University of Virginia School of Medicine and former secretary-general of the International League Against Epilepsy. Dr. Bertram told me I could have been having subclinical seizures at that time. This means that even though an epileptic seizure was unfolding, nothing felt or looked out of the ordinary to me or others around me. Dr. Bertram said sometimes those seizures can temporarily alter one's personality. In patients he has observed, some of their seizures aren't noticeable, but they have significant personality changes right after the seizure—everything from moodiness to major outbursts, paranoia to delusions. Sometimes those changes come the following day, and that's how people know they've had a seizure. In some people, the seizures could have been quietly happening for a long time.

My epileptologist, Dr. Winslow, agreed that it's possible for epileptic brain activity to affect mood even when seizures are not recognized. She told me that people can have behavior-type changes possibly noted before seizures too. This is called a prodrome, and it can happen a few hours or even a few days before the actual seizure. Common symptoms are anger and mood disorders, and they are common in temporal lobe epilepsy.

Then Dr. Winslow told me something that took me by huge surprise. There was a strong possibility that I truly was experiencing subclinical seizures, possibly dating back before that tonic-clonic seizure my junior year of college.

"It is common for those with seizures to have more subtle, less recognized seizures prior to having a bigger seizure, like you," she said.

That big seizure—the tonic-clonic—is a clinical seizure because there are visible symptoms like loss of consciousness and convulsing. Any change in behavior or feelings, like déjà vu, are also clinical seizures.

Once the clinical seizures went full-force, I had a feeling my new medication, Lamotrigine, was likely contributing to my irritability. Though the medication ironically is also used as a mood stabilizer, it can have other effects on people. The complexity of epilepsy is significant. It could be one thing or another driving the symptoms.

Without any of this knowledge at the time, I just assumed my medication was 100 percent at fault. At that point, controlling my seizures seemed easier than controlling my mood, as strange as that may seem. Keppra had caused mood swings in college, so I stopped taking it. Thankfully the seizures stayed at bay. Or at least I thought so, until hearing of the possibility that I could have been having silent seizures for four years.

I cut down my twice-daily dose of Lamotrigine a little, and then a little more. My moodiness decreased, but not by enough. Then I stopped taking Lamotrigine altogether. It wasn't known to me then that it takes a while for the body to get used to some antiseizure medications, but I didn't have a while. Adults need to control their emotions in the workplace, and I hated losing that control. But once I went off the medication, the seizures worsened.

One October afternoon, I joined coworkers at Sephora in a nearby mall to get makeovers for Heather's birthday. Heather told me that in the midst of the fun, the group heard a thud and turned around to see me flat on the floor.

Makeup would soon become my Band-Aid, a temporary fix to conceal my bruised eyes and cuts. Until I had more testing, which was the path Dr. Kiley was leading me down, I wouldn't have answers to what was causing the seizures. So far, I'd seen him twice in the clinic. His nurse continued to check in to ask how I was tolerating my medication and, of course, to ask if I was having seizures. I didn't tell her I had stopped the medication for a bit; I didn't want Dr. Kiley to get upset with me. But now it was obvious I needed to slowly build up my dose because I didn't want to try out a new ASM. If two had made me moody, would a third give me the same side effects? It felt like there was no time to start over, given my career goals, and I wasn't about to start taking a mood stabilizer. I wasn't aware of any coworkers who had a mental health condition, and so from where I sat, my fellow reporters were making easy progress on their way to larger television markets. They were pursuing my dream without any of my struggles. At the time, however, I didn't realize that my perspective wasn't necessarily accurate. I was too wrapped up in trying to hide seizures and their aftereffects to consider what others might be going through. The visibility of seizures made me assume everyone else's life was great.

So, for now, makeup covered my injuries and my insecurities, and like a Band-Aid, it was easy to reapply again and again should I fall on my face. Black-and-blue eyes faded to yellow-green bruises and eventually disappeared. It was as easy to brush on cheek blush as it was to brush off the seizures. I was denying the truth even while staring it in the face.

Perhaps if I had consciously experienced every seizure, my denial and resistance to changing my lifestyle would have softened. But at twenty-five years old, I simply wanted to be like my coworkers— healthy enough to do my job well without any accommodations and without any agony about whether, when, or where a seizure would strike.

It was lonely being an outsider, and I felt alone trying to navigate this unpredictable disease that was robbing me of a personal life and my memories. Nothing had challenged me this much. A bad race or a bad day at work was often a valuable experience for understanding what not to do the next time around. There was some reassurance in knowing that other reporters and athletes screwed up too. We could laugh at and curse those experiences.

But there was no comfort with epilepsy. No one I knew had seizures, and trying to explain my confusion during and after one was overwhelming and draining. At the time, I wasn't aware of the Epilepsy Foundation or support groups available to me, so I tried to fight through it on my own.

Determination and stubbornness fed this impossible belief that I was tough enough to get past seizures. Those traits had gotten me through everything else in life, so I stayed optimistic that my doctor would find the best dose of medication and that things would return to normal. But for these same reasons, I kept the news of my deteriorating health from my family. My parents knew I was seeing a neurologist for seizures, but I kept the details mostly in the dark. Still, my mom seemed to know something was up. I had a support system in place with friends and coworkers, and my family was seventeen hundred miles away, so it made the most sense—to me anyway—to wait to give them an update until I had the seizures under control.

Innocent phone calls and emails from very caring parents asking if I was feeling OK couldn't go unanswered, so why add more strain to my life? Or to theirs? It just made sense to hide the truth. But my parents had known me for twenty-five years, and I couldn't fool them. When I was writing this book, my mom told me she could tell from my deteriorating memory that I was having seizures back then.

But there was one person, thousands of miles away, whom I did confide in—Kara. She would listen but not tell me what to do. I simply wanted someone to hear me, not to advise.

"You were honest with me, always telling me about the seizures you had been having," she later told me. "You were very good at easing my worried mind by rationalizing. You would explain that the seizures were cause and effect (lack of sleep = seizures). I think I was under the impression at that time that the meds you were on were working."

My efforts to convince Kara that I was fine seemed to have worked.

After the seizure at Sephora, blood tests revealed to Dr. Kiley that I wasn't taking my medications as instructed. He documented his findings in my medical records:

10-4-10 "Would you call her and let her know that her Lamotrigine level is barely detectable. Is she taking it as I have instructed???"

11-22-10 "Lately I have been concerned that she is not too compliant."

Dr. Kiley increased my dose, and I started it again slowly, hoping my mood swings wouldn't return. So far, so good. I continued to take more to get up to the dose he prescribed. But more medication and fewer seizures couldn't control something that was slowly becoming more and more noticeable.

9

Missing Reminiscing

In the days and weeks following the seizures in 2010, I started waking up to the realization that bits and pieces of my life were . . . missing.

What did I do two weeks ago on my days off? And every weekend before that? What did Kara and Sara tell me on the phone last week?

Panic started creeping in.

Where did I get my oil changed? When was my last haircut or dentist appointment or seizure, and where? What did my family do for the holidays eight months ago? How am I forgetting seizures and nearly everything that happened on the day that one occurred?

At first, my memory loss seemed tied to the day of the seizure: most or all of that day would vanish. During the marathon in Seattle, slivers of the day remain intact, enough for me to reconstruct it. But most of the time, trying to recall a fun night, birthday, or race was like flipping through a photo album and only catching a glimpse of a single photo. Coming across that one photo stored deep in my brain brought both joy and sadness.

Thank you for holding onto a sliver of time, but why not two? Or five?

The concept of memory as something we can always have at our disposal is not always true. Epilepsy was slowly destroying my episodic memories of past and recent events—outings with my college roommates just five years prior, a road trip with coworkers one year prior, and news stories from just one month prior—but I usually didn't notice until people brought up a story. Time traveling through life events got murkier the further back I searched. Each time, my stomach sank in disbelief. In addition to episodic memory, my spatial memory started to decline—*How do I get to the grocery store again?* The only bright spot was that I wasn't forgetting important dates, such as my sister's birthday.

Eventually, huge periods of my life faded into the distance, including most of college, high school, and childhood. I was only twenty-five years old, and I couldn't remember college track meets, high school tennis meets, or my first job. Why? How?

Dr. Winslow told me that just like subclinical seizures can impact mood, they can affect memory in some patients even when no symptoms are present.

The other possible reason for my long-term episodic memory problems was simply the location the seizures were firing from. Various research shows that patients with unilateral temporal lobe pathology—meaning seizures that start in one temporal lobe— have greater loss of episodic than semantic autobiographical memories. The impairment stretches back to early childhood, far before seizures start.

I held onto the hope that someday I would be able to retrieve those early memories. But for now, I lived with the reality that having a career while living with epilepsy was like holding down two jobs—I was a news reporter for a local TV station and an investigative reporter in my own life. The latter became challenging work because I was uncomfortable asking questions about details of my life that I should already have known. Producing follow-ups to past stories at work soon also became very challenging because my working memory wasn't always working up to speed. I'd be talking with a coworker about a story I had done two days earlier and instantly lose my train of thought, like a passenger train flying off the tracks with no warning.

"I met with the superintendent about the budget and he explained why three, no wait, I think it was five . . . um . . . teachers would be furloughed . . . no wait, then he said it would be permanent . . . and . . ."

Nothing. My brain would go completely blank. A conversation that should have been seamless turned into a TV news story of flash frames.

Trouble with filling in the blanks during conversation soon had me forgetting names and faces or the order of events.

What news stories did I cover last week? After the Oregon Ducks feature but before the school board meeting?

About thirty seconds later, I'd make a quick retrieval.

Oh yeah, the one about the foreclosures. I did that story. But what was the story about?

Foreclosures made local and national news every week in 2010, but nothing struck a chord. For the next school board meeting, Eugene School District 4J discussed layoffs.

Did I interview the superintendent or a board member for that story?

Before the seizures worsened, my mind would do a quick rewind and pull up an image of the person in a few seconds. But it soon went from not remembering interviewees' faces to sometimes not remembering that I had interviewed them at all.

Searching for the big puzzle piece to connect everything together sometimes brought up nothing. Not even a hint. Without mental images of the interviewees and settings, my stories became a blank slate.

It was embarrassing to see someone I had spoken with or interviewed a few weeks earlier and then forget their name and face. Pretending became my go-to method. Smiling and listening intently for anything that might strike a chord sometimes did the trick, and I'd breathe a huge sigh of relief that I wouldn't need to bullshit my way through an entire conversation.

My memory deficits soon became annoying for my coworkers. Television news is fast-paced and unpredictable, and reporters need to remember past interviews because there's a good chance you'll do follow-ups, sometimes on short notice.

"Wait, when did that happen?" was not a good response when I was told to follow up on a story I had done previously, sometimes just weeks earlier. I tried hard not to ask questions.

A sharp memory is a huge advantage in this business because efficiency matters when a follow-up unfolds at four o'clock in the afternoon. The executive producer wants details plus a short refresher of the backstory for the five o'clock newscast. He then wants more details and a live shot at six, and if you work a nightside shift, he'll want all the details for a complete story at ten or eleven. I loved the adrenaline rush of working so quickly, but a memory block with the clock ticking would flatten me.

"C'mon Stacia," I'd mutter, snapping my fingers, drumming them on my desk, putting my hands on my chin, elbows on the table, and frantically searching the archives for my past scripts, even Googling them. Clocks were in every corner, on nearly every wall, and on my computer. There is no way to lose track of time in a newsroom.

My time in Eugene was the start of a long, slow downhill memory slide, both professionally and personally, as I grabbed for any and every clue possible to remind me of things I might have missed. Digital archives at work saved me more than once. Video footage would typically strike a chord, and often it was easier to recognize people's voices before their faces. Sometimes putting the face to the name brought some memories back, but other times it didn't.

Sometimes it was as if I had never done the news story to begin with. I imagine a good memory is like an internal calendar, one that people can easily flip through within a minute as the brain works in a frenzy to match up projects, holidays, birthday dinners, and sporting events. If a minute isn't enough time, it's easy to take out a planner or text a friend for the "Oh yeah, that's right!" moment.

Memory loss can be hard to quantify. How much should we be able to remember in life exactly? Comparing my memory bank to friends' was the best frame of reference. If they remembered our entire conversation from the month before, shouldn't I be able to as well? Or is memory based on how present we all were in the conversation? Maybe my memory of a situation is different from a friend's because we experienced it differently. I tried not to text or call people to fill in details unless it was urgent. Another reminder that I was young with a failing memory was defeating: the "Oh yeah, that's right!" moments were few and far between.

The few made my day.

Yay! I remembered my interviewee's name and the story from three weeks ago! Damn. I also remember who was sent home on *The Bachelor* that week. *Ugh, brain, get your priorities straight. Save room for the important stuff please.* I wondered if I remembered that night because laughing with friends took my mind off the seizures.

Not every laugh from those nights was saved, and that fact ruined my day.

Today, I only recall the winner of one episode.

Running helped me cope with the frustration and gave me space to breathe and smile again. Even if I couldn't train for races anymore, running four to thirteen miles on the trail tuned out the noise in my head.

My doctor recommended a journal to manage how I was tracking stories, conversations, and seizures. I scoffed at the idea after leaving his office.

You don't need a journal; focus harder during conversations and you'll be fine.

Denial was part of my reluctance. Why would I want to write down every seizure and admit that epilepsy was impacting so much of my life? Why would I want to remember the lowest points, like waking up to a stinging red mark from a hot iron that scalded my shoulder?

Ink is permanent on paper. A seizure is my eraser—there is no option to remember. But the damage is permanent.

That was the only positive thing about epilepsy—the bad stuff disappeared along with the good. With a journal, both would be visible. Anyone could find it, and although my roommate already knew about the seizures, what if I lost the journal when I eventually moved to my next job? What if my parents found it and discovered the seizures were far worse than I let on? Keeping everything locked up inside myself was safer. My problems were my problems, and I didn't want to revisit them.

I feared that anyone who read the journal would tell me that I had no business being a reporter anymore with my memory, that I would annoy people, would make too many mistakes, should find a different career. I didn't want a different career. Reporting hard news and producing solid, compelling features, meeting new people every day, and shooting and editing formed the perfect mix. I loved it. What else could I possibly do that would compare?

Looking back, I really wish I had compromised with myself and journaled two things: one, every seizure, so I could track the type and look for patterns with my sleep; and two, my favorite news stories and moments with friends and family. If I had known how much seizures would impact my memory long-term, I would have forced myself to jot down the things that made me smile. I would love to relive happy memories of my twenties today. The best of times would make me laugh and probably choke me up, but that's so much better than having just a blank slate.

////

"I don't remember."

I recognize the faces in the photo—Kate and Heather, my co-workers at KEZI. The gorgeous, pristine blue lake behind us is familiar because of its unique history. Crater Lake formed after a volcano erupted in central Oregon, and at almost two thousand feet, it's the deepest lake in the United States. Sunlight penetrates deep into the water, producing a color so intense it seems to pour right out of the photo.

Everyone says a picture is worth a thousand words. A single image can help us reminisce with family, friends, and coworkers. But living with epilepsy is like someone has taken a brush and with one swift stroke painted a thick black line straight through the events surrounding that wonderful moment. The photo of the three of us overlooking the water is right there on my computer. But staring at it doesn't bring me any closer to remembering that trip.

Was the hike hilly? How long was the drive? What did we eat and laugh about?

My brain wiped the entire day completely from my mind, leaving me not with a thousand words to describe the photo but three.

Three simple words that would become a familiar phrase for me, sometimes exasperating, sometimes embarrassing, and every time devastating.

"I don't remember."

The wide smile on my face is the only clue that I had a great time.

My best friend's wedding in our hometown is a blank slate, as is our backpacking adventure through Europe, my trip to Boston to see her, our road trip from Colorado Springs to Minnesota, and countless phone calls. Kara makes me laugh harder than anyone, and it hurts to know that hundreds of funny moments we shared are now forgotten to me. But she will recall them when we talk on the phone, and I'll start laughing all over again. Kara shared a moment she still cherishes from her wedding, telling me that I blew her away with a thoughtful, loving, heartfelt speech during the reception. I don't remember a single word from my speech or even a second of that day. It's one day I wish I could have back, to know why my words meant so much to her.

Wonderful life events, silly conversations, and fun experiences I've shared with friends and family are moments I treasure. Treasures are valuable and should be locked away, stored forever in our brains like a box of special photos in the attic, available to retrieve and reminisce over anytime. But both attics and brains are vulnerable to storms, and the damage can be minimal or catastrophic. The cause of my brainstorms was a mystery, which is the case for about 50 percent of people globally who have epileptic seizures, according to the World Health Organization.

Each second of déjà vu, each episode of jamais vu, and each flicker of light chipped away at my memory little by little, holiday by holiday, treasure by treasure.

The large Christmas tree, dressed in sparkling gold lights and delicate decorations, stood next to striped stockings hanging from our family's living room fireplace. The beautiful tree, dug out of the attic each December and planted on our hardwood floor, had been a consistent presence in our living room for twenty-five years.

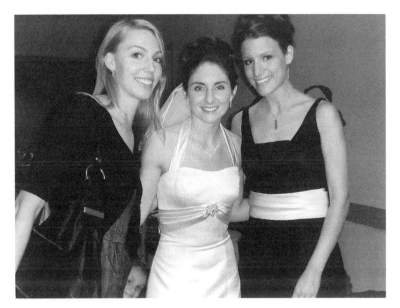

With my sister at Kara's wedding in 2009—one of many photographs showing an event I have no memory of.

Though I remember nearly every ornament placed over the years, I don't recall a single present that I wrapped or ripped open.

Hundreds of photos have piled up over the last fifteen years, each leaving me with questions: Who took the picture of me on a pier with waves crashing behind me? What is the story behind that photo of me on the sidelines at a Nebraska Huskers football game with a sports reporter, of my siblings and I on that ski hill, of me on a four-wheeler in the woods? Where was that indoor track meet and that photo with my teammates? When did I take that trip to Thief River Falls with Kara and to San Francisco to see Sara?

Photos don't always reveal the "who, what, where, and when," leaving me to wonder about everything except the "why." The "why" can be found in the facial expressions, often with a hint of laughter in bright, crinkled eyes.

Cameras can't always capture a thousand words, but they always capture a smile. And the size of mine tells me how much fun I was having in cities big and small across the Midwest and the West Coast. This was 2009 to 2011, when many people still used standard cameras and printed pictures. How I wish now that I would have written the location and event on the back of each photo and put together a few albums.

The purpose of life, I believed, was to live it fully, to explore what the world had to offer and share those experiences with others. Quality of life, then, is measured in those experiences but also in the small things, like great phone conversations. To completely forget about both within a week or a month or year later has been the hardest part of epilepsy, harder than the seizures themselves. Reminiscing with friends and family mostly brought up a blank space for me and disappointment and sadness in their eyes. They remembered the laughter, conversation, and food. They remembered the silly things I said and the serious things. The disbelief on their faces as they said "I already told you that" revealed that they felt unvalued, and I didn't blame them.

If I couldn't retain a memory, there was no option to recall, relive, or reminisce. Or, just as important, to reflect. Reflecting helps us learn from our mistakes and realize who we may have hurt. But what if you have a seizure and don't remember the mistake you made, who you hurt, or what you learned from it?

Forgetting feeds denial.

When did that seizure happen? I think maybe a few days ago? Couldn't tell you. I'm pretty sure I woke up by my bed. Not sure exactly. There are some bruises on my arm. Did I work that day? Well, it's all fine now.

Even though my seizures still weren't controlled, I kept my mouth shut over phone calls and emails to my family. I still assumed staying silent would worry them less. And I knew they would only tell me what I didn't want to hear. If the topic was on something I should have easily remembered, I avoided asking questions in order to reduce suspicion. But hiding the truth over the phone is much easier than in person. A challenge soon awaited me—my mom and brothers were coming to Oregon for a vacation.

Avoid asking any questions, I'd tell myself. They might repeat something they've said before, and you'll have to nod your head and pretend you remember. But my strategy would be impossible if they posed a question for me. I would have nowhere to turn.

You don't know what you have until it's gone. And until people ask you about it.

10

Level 4: Denial

In August 2011, nearly two years after I had moved to Eugene, my mom and my brothers, Mike and Tom, flew to Oregon. Our plan was to hike around Crater Lake, visit the coast, kayak, and visit Oregon Health and Science University (OHSU) in Portland. Tom and Mike were juniors in college at the time studying for careers in medicine, and they wanted to check out the campus.

But up first, wine. The day they arrived we decided to explore one of the state's many wineries, right outside Eugene.

My mom wanted to visit the same place I had taken her and my dad on their previous visit. There was one problem. I didn't know the name, the location, or that we had even visited a winery on their trip.

"You didn't know that you didn't know. As far as you were concerned, you were doing this for the first time," my mom recalled.

My mom was confused, and then it hit her. Seizures were the only explanation she could think of. She caught me. There was no way I could make up an excuse. Maybe for somebody in their eighties a memory lapse would be understandable, but not for me at twenty-six. The severity of my forgetfulness hit me in the face.

At work and with friends, I had sometimes been able to get away with forgetting small details, but not on a trip like this with my family there to bear witness.

I didn't know that I didn't know.

I had already visited that winery.

What was I supposed to say? How could I argue? Staying silent in that moment would show my weakness, show that I realized my problem was serious.

I couldn't do that.

I blew it off. Discussing seizures with my mom in front of my brothers would be agitating, and she didn't press the issue because she didn't want to ruin the trip for them.

But then it happened. Something I couldn't hide from her. During dinner, I went into the restroom to wash off a little food that had spilled on my shirt and had a small seizure at the sink. She wondered why I was gone so long just to blot a stain and grew suspicious.

"You came back to the table and admitted you had a seizure," she later told me.

Nobody mentioned my memory or that seizure for the rest of the trip, and I don't recall exactly what else we did; my brain erased every moment, and my mom filled in the blanks for me later. But I know we had fun. The last day brought an unexpected gift. If an undeniable problem with memory loss marked the start of the trip, it was only fitting that a potential solution would come at the end. It did, in the form of a flyer.

That morning we headed north to Portland to visit OHSU. Mike, Tom, and I jumped on a tram from the Center for Health & Healing to tour the medical school campus across the interstate. Mom stayed behind at the center's cafeteria. After a cup of coffee, she wandered around the lobby to kill time and came across a list of specialized departments next to the elevator. Upon first glance, "Brain Institute" caught her attention. She peered closer with interest and was surprised to see "OHSU Comprehensive Epilepsy Center."

The epilepsy center was also across the interstate, so she took the elevator up to the reception area to find out more. The doors opened, and a large kiosk with brochures caught her eye. She walked quickly over and sorted through the brochures to find the one on epilepsy and was amazed by the services offered there. Her excitement was clear as my brothers and I greeted her after touring campus.

"Stacia! I discovered there's a special center solely for epilepsy here! Here, look at this!"

"Really? Specialists for epilepsy?" I replied with surprise and curiosity, taking the brochure. "What do they do?"

The brochure stated the university had a level 4 epilepsy center. "What does that mean?" I wondered aloud.

"I found out there are four levels of epilepsy care, with level 4 being the highest," she explained.

We did a little digging and found that a full level 4 center has an epilepsy monitoring unit that is designed for inpatient stays of a few days or longer, with both EEG and video recording so doctors can observe and record patient seizures. The treatments available surprised me. Implants? Brain surgery? For seizures? Yikes!

OHSU was the closest level 4 epilepsy center to Eugene, a good two hours from my house, but going there for treatment wasn't possible since I couldn't drive. I kept the brochure though, hoping it might be helpful down the road, depending on where in the country I landed next.

Later that day, I hugged my mom and brothers goodbye before their flight, hoping my memory loss hadn't been too noticeable. But it had, and they boarded the plane more worried than ever.

Back at work, I shared the details of my fun weekend with Kate. But she was more interested in knowing if I had shared the extent of my seizures with my family. Kate had become a close friend in Eugene and was the person I confided in most.

"No, I didn't," I admitted. "I didn't want to frighten them."

She shook her head in disappointment, then later took the bold step of doing so herself. The correspondence between Kate and my mom makes clear the extent of my seizures and just how much I had been keeping my family in the dark.

September 15, 2011

Barb,

I am a good friend and co-worker of your daughter Stacia. I hope you and your family had a nice visit last month out to Oregon. . . . I'm not sure if you noticed a change in Stacia's health or memory when seeing her, but even though I've only known Stacia for less than 2 years, I've noticed her health dramatically downgrade in the past year.

I don't think that Stacia is coping well with the seriousness of her epilepsy. I think in part it is because the seizures wipe out her short-term memory, and she might not remember how many seizures she's actually had lately. One time we talked about her starting up a "seizure diary" so she could keep track but I don't think she ever implemented that idea.

I've been with Stacia multiple times when she's had seizures, and I don't think she's upfront with me, her friends, her boss, or even her family on how often she suffers from them. But she often shows up to work with bruises, scrapes, and injuries from times she's collapsed at home. I know she is fiercely independent, and loves her job, her freedom and her health, but it worries me that she's not telling her doctor or her family how often she has seizures and how much her condition is affecting her life. . . .

Stacia told me all weekend long last weekend she had many seizures. I asked if she was going to tell her doctor, and she said no. She often blames her seizures on not getting enough sleep, but I wonder if that is her way of dealing with the mystery of not understanding her condition, and thus not being proactive about finding treatment. I am concerned for her health and well-being. And I just want her to get the medical attention she needs, and I believe she needs to be held accountable by people that love and care for her.

Kate

/ / / /

September 15, 2011

Kate, thank you so much for your message.

I'll be forever grateful that you contacted me. I worry about Stacia 24/7 and live in constant fear that something will happen to her. Independent she is! She shut me out from my inquiries about her condition long ago, but I know her life has changed. She rarely speaks about going out anymore and seems to sleep every spare moment she has. My first reaction is to see if she could get a medical leave of absence and come home where I can watch her on a daily basis until she finds a set of meds that work for her. . . .

Could I ask for your advice? I'm not sure where to turn—call her doctor? Come out to Oregon and get her? As a mom, I wish she were 16 instead of 26 so I had some legal control! I go into the station's website daily to see if she made it to work.

Barb

Kate encouraged my mom to come to Oregon in early October to meet with my doctor. My mom knew she would have to break the news of their visit to me eventually—and that I wouldn't be happy about it—but because I rarely shared news of my seizures with my parents, she also asked Kate for some background and a little history about my seizures.

September 16, 2011

Barb,

I am so glad to hear that you are coming out for a week and will get to meet with Stacia's doctor. I expect Stacia will be really upset, but my hope and prayer is that in the end she'll realize how serious living with this condition is.

I don't have any idea how often Stacia has seizures. But Heather and I were estimating that it's up in the hundreds . . . this year. Because oftentimes her seizures come in series where she has a couple small seizures after the big one . . . and some "small seizures" are likely her being confused in the recovery period. Last winter she had a seizure on-air while interviewing the mayor. . . . She fell at the station, and then had them all weekend long. She has admitted to having seizures while sitting at the edit bays at work. I think they are less physical and more of her brain shutting down. She's told me that she's had them in the shower and on runs.

Heather says she's been on several live shots or stories with Stacia where she's had them. And one time she had them while interviewing someone, so she asked Heather to take over. After the Seattle marathon she had seizures all weekend long at home. She often shows up to work with mysterious injuries: black eyes, a brick print on her head, cuts on her arms, a burn on her shoulder from falling into an iron. I'm sorry if this list is startling to you. And even just compiling this list made me realize I should have written this email long ago. Let me know if you have any other questions. Thanks for being such a good mom to Stacia!

Kate

My mom was curious about how I reacted to the seizures when Kate and others were with me. She asked whether I have tears in my eyes, whether I get upset or make excuses. In her words, "Tears would mean she wants help. Excuses means she doesn't." My mom knew I wanted to continue working in television journalism and said that goal alone should be enough to make me face the severity of my epilepsy. Kate rarely saw me shaking when I had a seizure and said I would usually wake up confused and disoriented. Sometimes she'd hear me curse in a very disappointed tone. The news was all my mom needed to hear, and she assured Kate that my dad would call me and break the news of their plans to visit.

I don't remember who called, or the conversation, but I know I wasn't pleasant. At first, my anger was directed toward whoever at work had contacted my mom. She wouldn't tell me.

Was it Sean? He was the assistant news director and saw me every day.

Who else? Kate?

At the time, my mom didn't confirm her identity or tell me what was in the emails, but I had a strong feeling Kate had written them. The news provoked both anger and surprise. Would I ever have the guts to tell a coworker's mom that her daughter wasn't taking care of her health? No. That was gutsy. At the time, I felt betrayed. But now, years on, I'm impressed with Kate. We'd known each other only a year and a half when she sent those emails. Nothing would stop my parents from coming to Eugene, and my siblings were very much on their side. Bitterly, I agreed to schedule an appointment with Dr. Kiley on the soonest day that both their calendars could match up. Eighteen days later, they arrived.

"We knew it would be very unpleasant for us," my mom later told me, "and it was."

I have no memory from that day, so my parents recounted the conversation we had at a local restaurant.

"You were upset, insisting that we didn't need to have come out. You kept saying that you were figuring out your medication dose with your doctor," my dad told me.

"I told you pretty sternly that you needed to understand that we are your parents and care about you," my mom added. "Your condition belongs to our entire family, and you need to let us in on this. The decisions you make affect all of us and we shouldn't have to wait for a friend to tell us things are much more serious than what you've led us to believe on the phone."

Her tone didn't surprise me. We had been raised to be independent from an early age and had worked part-time to earn spending money. It was understood that we would be expected to put ourselves through college and that we should spend time considering what we wanted to study and how we would pay off our loans.

That independent mentality stayed with me but proved detrimental once epilepsy entered my life. My strong reaction to my parents' visit is something I now regret, but at the time, I wasn't seeking attention. I was twenty-six years old and I didn't want anyone pressing me with questions or to hear the words "We're really worried about you." I didn't want them to question me when I said, "I'm fine," because I knew what they would ask next.

Fine with what, Stacia?

Fine with worrying loved ones and coworkers?

Fine with banging up a head that's already scarred and having seizures?

Fine with forgetting simple conversations and weekends with your friends?

I was fine with it all, because I believed it was my problem to deal with, nobody else's. Coworkers were starting to make career jumps, and I didn't want to let seizures stand in my way.

My entire family would insist on more in-depth testing, but that would require trips to the epilepsy center at OHSU in Portland. I would have felt like a burden asking anyone to drive me the two hours there and back. The cost of medical care was the other issue. Hospitals and neurology clinics in Portland were out of network. My deductible was already high enough, and fees didn't stop once the deductible was met. The logical choice was to remain in Eugene, stay the medication course, and move to a city with a bigger neurology center once my contract was up.

The situation felt impossible. How many months would it take for doctors to figure out my seizures and find the correct medication dose? What if they couldn't? How could I get back into TV news if I took time off for treatment? How would I get health insurance?

Insurance already didn't cover one of my medications, so what else would they deny? Who would hire me if I didn't have any recent work to show?

Legally, I knew employers couldn't ask questions about medical conditions, but a simple peek at the time gap would raise a red flag.

Should I put my career above my health? Or my health above my career?

My parents and I met with Dr. Kiley the next day. Memory problems surfaced yet again once we arrived at the clinic, and I don't recall anything from that day.

"You had no idea where his office was, even though you'd been there before," my dad told me later. "Mom and I followed you around until we finally stopped to ask for directions. That was very tough on us to see you like that."

Once a nurse led us into a small clinic room, there really was nowhere for me to hide, no more excuses to make. My mom had witnessed a few seizures and could clearly see the impact of my memory loss during her short visit with my brothers. I was too wrapped up in my disappointment about forgetting where Dr. Kiley's office was to consider how stressful it must have been for my parents. Their oldest daughter had little recollection of every important moment they had been a part of, including her childhood and most of high school.

After we sat down with Dr. Kiley, I gave him an update. At that point, I was taking a higher dose of medication and tolerating it much better. The wild mood swings had stopped. Was Lamotrigine now preventing some subclinical seizures? Or did my brain just need to adjust to the medication?

But I told him I was still suffering seizures and usually losing awareness.

"I'm concerned about her sleep. And I wonder if she's having more seizures than she is aware of," my mom told Dr. Kiley.

He had written a similar opinion in my medical notes following an earlier appointment: "I would wonder if Stacia is under more stress than she lets on. She has a tendency to downplay or deny aspects of her physical and mental health."

Dr. Kiley told my parents he wasn't allowed to share anything I wouldn't give him permission to, because I was a legal adult. But according to my dad, that didn't stop him from speaking rather bluntly to me about taking my situation more seriously.

My mom summarized our discussion with Dr. Kiley in an email:

You agreed to tell me about any new seizures and share medical updates.

Here is the deal we made when Dad and I visited you:
You promised to be a good patient. This means:

1. You will let your doctor decide on your treatment, not you. Thus, he gets to decide on your meds. You will let him know the side effects of your meds so he can adjust them accordingly. He said that he will keep

trying meds until he finds one that (1) you can tolerate and (2) will leave you seizure free.

2. You will call your doctor after each seizure so he can work with you. He can't do his job without this information.

3. You will keep me informed.

I promised:

To pay for your neurology related bills so you won't use this as an excuse to not work with your doctor. As discussed, this is a small price to pay for your health and my peace of mind.

Remember, this disease isn't yours alone, it belongs to your family, friends and everyone who loves you.

I trust you will keep your end of the deal, Stacia. Don't let me down.

With that said, my mind continues to reflect on what your siblings and Kate said. *Sara*: all this happened in Eugene but when she gets her new job, she will start fresh. *Tom*: Stacia has been successful in everything she's done. She now needs to find success with this disease. *Mike*: she needs to go to the best place in the U.S. to get this taken care of. *Kate*: she needs to be responsible to those who love her.

Please print this and glue it to your nose.

This was the first time I'd seen my siblings' and Kate's feelings together at one time.

Everyone wanted the best for me. I knew that. But seeing healthy people in their early twenties tell someone with uncontrollable seizures that she needed to do this and needed to do that put me on edge.

It sounds so simple, doesn't it?

But the fact that everyone I loved was on the same page—literally—meant that ignoring any of them wasn't an option. Kate made that clear. The rest of the email seemed fair enough. Mom made me realize that parents worry a lot, but she worried even more after the bare-bones updates I shared from halfway across the country. The more I talked, she said, the less she would fret. That had been the opposite of my thinking, but I didn't have kids, and I couldn't argue.

In retrospect, I wish I had been less stubborn and more agreeable and grateful that my parents were flying halfway across the country on short notice to help me. Controlling seizures needed to be my priority, and my mom was determined that I would see it too. I also wish I hadn't shooed away coworkers and friends. Kate saw my epilepsy spiraling out of control and my insistence on putting my job above my health. I never thought to ask my neurologist if there were support groups; years later I found out that the Epilepsy Foundation hosts them in multiple states.

One week after the appointment with my parents, I was back with Dr. Kiley for a thirty-seven-minute awake/asleep EEG to try to identify where the seizures were originating from. The results were not much different from the findings in my medical notes at the University of Minnesota: "Fairly unremarkable awake and asleep EEG other than two subtle episodes of right temporal disorganization and slowing."

Temporal slowing means that the brain waves are traveling at a slower frequency than normal. It was clear to me by then that neurological diseases are challenging to treat because the human brain is so complex. The outcome once again made me optimistic that maybe I didn't really have epilepsy but still disappointed there wasn't a clear reason for my seizures. I knew deep down that a more advanced epilepsy center was in my future.

Thank you, Mom, for finding out about level 4 epilepsy centers.

11

Looking for Answers

My two-year contract at the station in Eugene was nearing an end. The timing felt perfect; armed with the knowledge about level 4 epilepsy centers, I would prioritize finding a top-tier medical center while searching for my next job. The United States is home to around 115 level 4 epilepsy centers, and most are concentrated in larger metro areas. I hoped my career would land me near one.

The cards matched up perfectly. Grand Rapids, Michigan, had a job opening for a news reporter and was home to two level 4 epilepsy centers. It was a stroke of luck to have access to great medical care in Grand Rapids so I wouldn't have to travel to Ann Arbor, Lansing, or Detroit. Saying goodbye to my Oregon coworkers was hard; they had been such a fun group to work with. But many of them would soon take off for their next career moves too. Kate and another coworker, Susan, would take jobs in the Twin Cities, so I got to see them again on trips home.

Starting off 2012 with a new reporting adventure and new medical care had me optimistic that Michigan was the right move. Once my benefits kicked in, I made an appointment first with a primary care physician to get a referral for neurology. One of the level 4 epilepsy centers in Grand Rapids had recently opened. Spectrum Health Butterworth Hospital's (now Corewell Health's) Epilepsy Monitoring Unit housed inpatient rooms with EEG and video recording. Two epileptologists who led the epilepsy program at Henry Ford Hospital in Detroit came to Grand Rapids to open the unit.

One of the doctors was Dr. Brien Smith, the board chair of the Epilepsy Foundation at the time, a national organization that serves people with epilepsy. I called the hospital in hopes of seeing whichever doctor had the first available appointment and was told

Dr. Smith could see me in six months. I was disappointed but figured six months would be worth the wait. My seizures were thankfully under control for now, and I was very intent on keeping them that way. With improved sleep, I truly believed I could join the majority of people whose seizures are controlled long-term. The excitement of a new start gave me energy to pack up my stuff quickly and ship everything to Michigan so I would be ready to start my new job right away in January.

An alarm ringing insistently at 2:00 a.m. would be part of my new routine. I was hired to be the new morning reporter at a local TV station in Grand Rapids, similar to the shift I had worked in Eugene. The unpleasant blare of the alarm bolted me out of bed with a groan. Every work shift started around 3:30 a.m. to prepare for live shots for the 5:00 a.m. and 6:00 a.m. newscasts. On a typical morning, I would report live a few times, then start making phone calls for a different story for the following day. But the entire day could change in a second if there was breaking news. Sometimes I worked with a photographer; at other times I was shooting, writing, and editing my own stories.

I left work around 12:30 p.m. each day, still energized, and hoped to be in bed by 6:00 p.m., but it was often a struggle to fall asleep that early, especially in the summer with more hours of sunlight. I managed to keep my brain calm during work. But it would rebel at night and on weekends. My sleep improved with the aid of medication, so I stuck to a 6:00 p.m. bedtime in order to get in a run before work.

Even though I became more comfortable discussing seizures with friends in Oregon, I had zero plans to tell anyone in Michigan. This would be a new start, and I knew only one person at the new station. At twenty-seven, I was one of the youngest reporters on staff. In Oregon, it was reassuring to have friends and coworkers who knew exactly what my seizures looked like and what to do if I had one. Going into work each day and not having to hide a serious, unpredictable brain disease took some of the pressure off. And it was nice to know people cared. I figured I couldn't be diagnosed for sure without real tests in Grand Rapids, so why tell my new friends? I didn't know enough about seizures to answer every question they may have had. You might call that denial, but my perspective was, hey, I had seizures in Oregon, but Michigan so far has been a smooth ride. I would stay on my medication and dedicate my life to sleep for the next six months until my new doctor could evaluate me. It worked. Seizures stayed away.

Finally, the day arrived. Six months after moving to Grand Rapids, I finally met my new epileptologist, Dr. Brien Smith. He greeted me with a big smile and handshake, and his easygoing demeanor and friendliness calmed my nerves right away. He added the anti-seizure medication Zonisamide to my dose of Lamotrigine and scheduled a two-hour EEG for the following week.

The upcoming EEG dominated my thoughts all week. My three previous EEGs from the University of Minnesota and Oregon had not provided any concrete answers, and I so hoped the fourth would do it. I stayed positive as I walked back into Butterworth Hospital, because dwelling on the EEG wouldn't change the outcome. My brain would do whatever it wanted to do for the next two hours. And, as it turned out, it stayed calm. The EEG recorded no electrographic seizures, nor did doctors see any clinical seizures.

My confidence rose—maybe I didn't really have epilepsy after all. Maybe something else was wrong. But Dr. Smith reminded me that a two-hour EEG didn't mean I was in the clear. A 24/7 video EEG was up next, in the hospital's epilepsy monitoring unit (EMU). The EEG would once again record brain waves, while a video camera would capture all my behavior. Round-the-clock testing for three to seven days usually gives doctors enough material to make a good diagnosis and consider further treatments, though not always. The next EMU opening was three months out. The timing couldn't have been better.

////

Expect the unexpected—reporters and distance runners alike learn to live by this rule. In the news business, a story can change on a dime. And in running, the marathons in Lincoln and Seattle proved I didn't know how my body would react under racing stressors. But more so than careers and sports, and more so than most medical conditions, "expect the unexpected" could be the slogan for epilepsy. People wake up every day wondering if a seizure might strike at the worst possible moment. I tried to avoid the image of myself during an aura, but it followed me everywhere if I didn't get enough rest.

It's harder to accept the unknown. But I hoped the EMU results would give me more peace of mind and help me learn how to expect the unexpected.

Finally, in November 2012 an EMU room opened. My mom traveled from northwest Minnesota to join me, and we stayed at my apartment the night before the epilepsy study. I don't remember her visit, but that evening she discovered something I never could have known on my own. She told me that when dinner ended, I headed down the hall to brush my teeth while she started washing the dishes. As she was scrubbing a plate, a loud thud jolted her upright. She headed quickly toward the bathroom and found me on the ground, face up with my toothbrush in my mouth.

My mom said I was out for about fifteen seconds.

She was puzzled because I hadn't moved an inch once I fell, which isn't what she would have expected with a seizure. She said I quickly came to and released the toothbrush from my mouth. Neither of us knew what could have caused this.

The episode left me perplexed. I had gotten dizzy brushing my teeth and washing my face in the past and had sometimes blacked out. Those were what I called my "tiny seizures." There was never an aura with those episodes, which was uncommon for me. But how many times did I actually fall to the floor during them?

Not enough times to remember.

Had this episode been a drop seizure, where people lose some or all muscle tone and abruptly drop to the floor? Those seizures last around fifteen seconds.

The answers would come soon enough.

The next day, on a chilly late November morning, my mom and I arrived at Spectrum Health Butterworth Hospital and headed to

the Epilepsy Monitoring Unit. A nurse led us down the white hallway to my room, which was fairly standard for a hospital setting—
bed, chair, TV, bathroom—with the exception of a few things. A
small black dome on the wall caught my eye; the video camera
would roll twenty-four hours a day to capture seizures in my bed
or wherever I moved in the room. Audio recording would distin-
guish if I was yelling, mumbling, or talking incoherently during
the seizures. Bumper pads cushioned my bed rails to prevent me
from hurting or breaking limbs if I started kicking my legs or convulsing. Thankfully, the nurses would allow me to walk around a
little during the study. Then, to the side of the bed, on the ground,
were pedals, like those on a stationary bike.

Once I settled into my room, an EEG technician arrived with the
familiar kit containing electrodes.

"Ah, I'm used to this by now," I smiled.

Multiple wires hung from my head like thin braids before the
technician secured them under a helmet of gauze and tape. The
wires connected to the EEG machine, and moments later, my brain
waves appeared in a steady rhythm, the video camera above my
head started rolling, and the waiting game began.

The plan was to gradually reduce my medications and deprive
me of sleep to increase the chance that my neurons would misfire.
Patients can stay in the room and be monitored for up to a week,
in certain cases even longer, but if enough seizures take place
early in the study, they are released sooner. This was one time I
really wanted to have seizures, to get Dr. Smith the information he
needed so I could get out of the hospital quickly. A nurse handed
me a little button to press if I felt a seizure coming on and secured
an IV for immediate access to medication to stop a prolonged seizure. Rescue medication, now that was a scary concept.

*This meant one of my seizures might start and not stop? Well, at
least a bed outfitted with bumper pads and a safety belt was a safe place
to find out.*

Next came a few more sticky electrodes for my chest, with wires
hooked to a different monitor. My heart rate popped up on the
screen. EEG and cardiac telemetry combined would monitor all

electricity in my brain and heart. I settled in, trying to distract myself from what I sort of hoped, yet dreaded, would come: flashing light hallucinations, déjà vu, jamais vu, or whatever other strange symptoms would provide the answers we needed. Reading and phone calls with friends would keep my mind off my brain. That was the plan anyway. By around 12:30 p.m., it was time for lunch.

I have no recollection of what happened next, but the video recording shows it clearly.

Notes from my medical record stated, "She was noted during EEG to have abnormal activity, including putting her hand over her face indicating she did not feel well. She was asked what was wrong and started blinking frequently but was unable to describe what was happening."

Then my eyes closed, and I went completely still for seven seconds. Five hours later the unexpected behavior returned, only worse. As I sat at the side of my bed, the camera caught me blinking frequently again, all while my heart rate started a slow decline for seventeen seconds. Then, my heart paused for thirteen seconds. My head dropped and I collapsed on my side.

Were these drop seizures? The EEG only showed generalized polyspike discharges, but my medical team said they couldn't confirm the spikes were associated with epilepsy. Meanwhile, the cardiac telemetry didn't show waves at all during those seven-second and thirteen-second pauses, but instead a flat line. I had fainted twice. My recovery time was much quicker than a typical seizure, mirroring what my mom had seen the night before at my apartment. She said I had some confusion, but it passed quickly.

Finding the source of my seizures was no longer the immediate priority. At 6:30 p.m. doctors wheeled me over to the Meijer Heart Center and called in a cardiac surgeon. Confusion swirled in my tired brain. The questions now were obvious even to me:

Were some of the seizures actually seizures, or had I been fainting?

Can seizures cause heart arrhythmias?

Can heart arrhythmias cause seizures?

Or did I have two unrelated health problems? And if so, why

would they come into my life and create havoc at the same time? That seemed like too much of a coincidence.

My heart would provide some answers first.

An EEG machine followed me to the heart center to keep an eye out for any misfiring neurons. Dr. Vinayak Manohar arrived and determined that a temporary pacemaker was necessary, so at 10:00 p.m. he inserted a sheath—a plastic tube—into a large vein in my right thigh. The sheath guided a wire up to my heart, then Dr. Manohar connected the other end to an external pacemaker.

Over the next forty hours that leg had to lie motionless on the hospital bed while the pacemaker recorded my heart pausing again and again. That's nearly two days without moving a limb even an inch! To go from rushing around all day at work with my camera or exercising to lying completely still was a true lesson in patience. And that was also nearly two days without a single spike or seizure recorded on the EEG, which was a stroke of luck. My body did not sit still during seizures. I didn't want to even think about what could have happened with that wire in my leg if a seizure had struck.

A nurse peeked in often to remind me not to let my leg move. All the motionless hours on end gave Dr. Manohar the information he needed. The diagnosis was sick sinus syndrome, essentially a sick heart. The sinus node, located in the upper chamber, is the heart's natural pacemaker because it controls the heartbeat by giving it a steady pace of electrical impulses. But my heart was only beating 32 bpm on average and occasionally taking breaks. Sounded to me like an out of shape runner. The condition is uncommon and mostly affects the elderly.

Dr. H. Paul Singh inserted a permanent pacemaker to prevent any more pauses. I had completely forgotten about the Holter heart study and bradycardia diagnosis in college. This slow heart rate stuff was old news, but it was brand-new to me in Michigan. So was the fainting.

Why hadn't doctors given me a pacemaker back then?

It was because I had been asymptomatic—I never got dizzy or fainted. Many endurance athletes have slow heart rates because they're in great shape and never have any issues. That had been me seven years earlier.

When did things change?

No one knows. The new pacemaker set my heart rate at 60 bpm, 24/7. The pacemaker acted as insurance—it would only pace my heart if it started to slow down and would kick it into motion if it took a break.

So, I fainted twice during my first day at the hospital, rebounding quickly, and the EEG didn't show any definitive seizure activity. My mom told my doctor the exact same scenario had played out in my apartment. And most of the "tiny seizures" I was having prior to this hospitalization happened while washing my face and brushing my teeth. Had I been fainting all along? Was bending down over the sink causing me to faint?

Suddenly my mind flooded with questions as I tried to piece together what had happened.

If this was happening repeatedly in the hospital, was my heart pausing day-to-day at work and on the running trail?

Auras sometimes gave me a few seconds to sit down, but not the dizziness.

Maybe the fainting could explain some of the black-and-blue marks, but how long had this been happening? A flashback appeared of a recent incident in my Michigan kitchen. I had woken up on the floor next to my kitchen cabinet with a throbbing foot. That one had to have been a tonic-clonic seizure because I must have kicked something to hurt my foot. But EEG testing down the road would reveal the kicking could have been a much different type of seizure.

But how is it that I never fainted at work? Surely someone would have noticed.

The possibility raised my heart rate slightly in excitement.

Maybe I don't have epilepsy! Maybe my heart is responsible for the seizures and the pacemaker will solve everything!

My hopes were high when Dr. Smith stopped by to check on me. He shook his head with an apologetic smile.

"I think you still do have epilepsy."

So the electrical systems in both my heart and my brain were screwed up. My spirits sank.

Why? What's responsible for all the power outages? How could both problems have shown up unannounced in college, then seemingly quieted down, and now suddenly started failing at the same time?

What happened to my once healthy body?

Now that I had the safety net of the pacemaker, I was less worried and more curious about a possible correlation. How could the two most important parts of the body—the brain and the heart—create problems for each other? At this point, doctors didn't know what was causing the seizures, nor how long my sinus node had been sick.

The pacemaker solved one problem. As for the other, only time would tell. I had gone to the hospital for one problem and walked out with two.

If the doctors hadn't found the issue with my heart, I don't know where I would be today.

Dates are easy to lose track of in the hospital, but I knew this was a Thursday. I had been home in Minnesota for Thanksgiving exactly a week before, reflecting on all the things I was thankful for, like my upcoming epilepsy testing. My admission date was Monday, and here I was four days later. Thanksgiving Day had turned into Thanksgiving week.

I don't know how long my heart could have held up under the daily cycle of pause/restart/pause/restart. Seizures had likely saved my life; sick sinus syndrome usually worsens over time, and my doctors may not have ever caught the heart issue if I hadn't bothered to treat my seizures.

"Go home and rest up, and we'll get you back in here for the EEG study before the holidays," Dr. Smith instructed.

I was full of gratitude as I left the hospital. Thanksgiving 2012 is my most memorable one to date. Talk about a reason to be thankful. How's that for expecting the unexpected?

Now back to the real world, where the new test would begin.

How many of my so-called seizures were in fact fainting?

Knowing that running was my trigger for seizures made me more curious about whether it was also affecting my heart.

I was both hesitant and impatient to find out.

A few days after leaving the hospital, my feet were ready to hit the pavement. Bedrest is hard on a body. Six days after my release, I bent down to tie my shoes and felt myself gasp. I couldn't breathe in; it was as if a vacuum was sucking the air out of my lungs. My chest immediately tightened, and I fought for air. Confused and a little frightened, I stood up and let my breathing return to normal. Since it did so quickly, I shrugged it off and headed down the stairs and out the door to run. My symptoms disappeared once my arms started pumping, and I felt fine the rest of the day. The same pattern followed the second morning. I again brushed it off because the symptoms disappeared on my run. But that didn't last long. I went into work and remember getting dizzy while walking up a small hill on a bridge during my story. Luckily, a videographer was working with me because I was restricted from driving and lifting camera gear following the pacemaker surgery.

My symptoms subsided enough that I was able to go back to the news station, log my video, and write the story for the evening newscast. Then it was time to do my voiceover. I walked across the newsroom and into the edit room with my script, set up the computer, and hit the record button. Only one sentence in, my lungs were gasping for air. I stopped the recording and just stood there for a few seconds.

Breathe . . . you're fine . . . take a deep breath . . . slow down and relax.

Voicing a news story requires more breath and energy than talking in a typical conversation. After calming myself down, I hit record a second time. Once again, I couldn't catch my breath. My friend and coworker Sarah was voicing her story in the booth next to me and sensed something was wrong. She knocked on my door and let herself in.

"Stacia, I could hear you through the wall; you sounded short of breath," she said with concern. "You need to go to the hospital." Her voice was firm.

"No, I need to finish the story first or our producers will be scrambling to fill my spot," I said back stubbornly, forcing the words out. "I'm fine."

I turned my shoulders back to the mic, took a big breath to calm down, hit record, and attempted to push the words out of my mouth. My lungs rebelled and I started hyperventilating.

"You're going to the hospital. I'm going to get the news director," Sarah said and left quickly without giving me a chance to respond.

Meanwhile, I calmed down and left the audio booth to call my cardiologist, who instructed me to get an X-ray immediately. I figured a trip to the emergency room wasn't necessary for an X-ray, so my friend and coworker Alana drove me across town to an urgent care clinic. My symptoms upon walking in hadn't improved.

"Chest pain and shortness of breath," I told the nurse. The X-ray showed that the pacemaker was in place but revealed nothing else. The other test I needed at that point couldn't be done at an urgent care clinic, so they ordered me to head to the ER.

Sarah picked me up, but I didn't want to go. She was concerned and irritated, and looking back, I don't blame her.

"Why are you being so stubborn?" she asked.

There were a few reasons: I had already missed almost a week of work and even at age twenty-seven I still thought I was a little invincible. My doctors discovered a heart problem and had taken care of it, so what else could possibly go wrong? All I knew is that it was dinner time, I was hungry, and we had planned to attend a work gathering that had already started, so we stopped and got food.

The minute we finished eating Sarah ordered me out the door, and we soon pulled up to the ER of the same hospital that had released me the week before. Doctors ordered a CT of my chest to rule out a pulmonary embolism—a clot that stops blood flow to an artery in the lung. The results came back quickly, and the doctor looked very serious as she turned to show me the CT scan image of my lungs.

"You're lucky you came in tonight," she said.

There were pulmonary emboli in both lungs. I knew nothing about blood clots other than that they were bad news. The doctor admitted me, and before long I was tying on a faded blue gown, sliding into fuzzy hospital slippers, and holding out my arm for a nurse to insert an IV. Heparin would drip into my veins for the next two days to dissolve the clots. Too restless to sleep in a hospital bed, my mind started to replay the week that had led me here.

Eleven days earlier, epilepsy monitoring had revealed a heart arrhythmia that could have eventually killed me. Treating sick sinus syndrome required two days of immobility and extreme concentration; my leg couldn't move an inch with the temporary pacemaker inserted. As a result, blood wasn't circulating as quickly as it should. That put me at risk for a deep vein thrombosis, a blood clot that starts in a leg vein, breaks off, and usually ends up in one or both lungs. That's exactly what happened. I had been given a blood thinner but it must not have been enough to prevent the clot.

Sarah and Alana no doubt saved my life that day. Lesson learned—I shouldn't have downplayed my shortness of breath, especially following surgery.

In a way, running also saved my life. The warning signs had appeared while bending down to tie my shoes. The irony hit me— my brain usually hates running. It triggers seizures. But in this instance, running had alerted me to an acute medical problem that needed immediate attention.

When Dr. Smith stopped by my hospital room, he said something that ended up changing the course of my life. He had decided not to do the epilepsy video EEG for eight more months, until I was off warfarin, a blood thinner.

Getting that news felt as if a balloon that had slowly filled with hope since moving to Michigan had just popped. The waiting game, the daily questioning if my seizures could be cured, would start all over again. I was crushed. Dr. Smith wanted to trigger seizures, and the chance of me falling during a seizure and potentially suffering internal bleeding while on a blood thinner was too risky.

I wanted more than just answers about my brain—I also wanted to avoid an entire year of health insurance costs again. The pacemaker surgery used up my deductible and out-of-pocket maximum payment for 2012, which ate up a big chunk of my salary that year. Treatment of the pulmonary embolism was covered and the epilepsy study in December would have been too. Now waiting until 2013 meant starting all over with expensive hospital bills.

Good health is a gift not only for quality of life.

Just take it one week at a time, I told myself.

12

Bizarre and Unique

Spectrum Health Medical Records, by Brien Smith, MD
2nd Round EMU—August 2013
Spectrum Health Butterworth Hospital, Epilepsy
Monitoring Unit
Clinical seizure description:
"Bizarre Complex Partial Seizures"

Eight long months later, the blood clots were a distant memory, and hopefully the doctors could determine the reason behind my memory loss. Did I have temporal lobe epilepsy like my Oregon neurologist Dr. Kiley had diagnosed?

What eventually unfolded was surprising even to my doctors.

A nurse walked me down the same hallway as my last EMU visit and into a familiar room. Epilepsy Monitoring Unit, take 2. Onto my scalp and chest went the electrodes, and into my hand came the seizure alert button. Telemetry would monitor my heart. Compression sleeves and Lovenox would keep blood clots away. Sleep deprivation and reducing my ASM would hopefully trigger seizures.

The cards were in place, and the waiting game began once again. The first night my dad offered to stay up all night to keep me company. He had driven fifteen hours from Thief River Falls and was tired but still tried to keep me awake. I was grateful for the support and for someone to talk with. My parents were amazing, though I didn't appreciate all the sacrifices they made during that stretch of my life.

The sleep deprivation worked. My first seizure—and the first my dad had ever seen—struck around seven o'clock in the morning, right as I was digging into breakfast.

"You spaced out as you started eating cereal and then turned the bowl over and dumped it out," he told me.

Well, that's embarrassing. Seizures can throw all things rational out the window. Typically, neurons fire in a consistent pattern, so we make good judgment calls and can follow social norms, like not dumping cereal on a hospital floor. That's when the brain is in balance.

But during a seizure, multiple neurons send signals simultaneously and much faster than usual. This surge of electrical activity scrambles messages in the brain.

If the seizure also alters the person's consciousness, any number of unusual behaviors can unfold. It's a frightening thought—even scarier when it plays out in an instant.

The EEG didn't pick up the seizure activity this time, and it wouldn't for some of the other small episodes in the following days. But Dr. Smith said that didn't rule out epileptic seizures. If a seizure forms deep inside the temporal lobe, and therefore farther away from the electrodes, the EEG might not pick it up.

Thankfully my dad didn't have to witness what was to come later in the week.

Day 2, no seizures.

C'mon brain, do your job so I can get out of the hospital at some point.

On day 3, a seizure struck at 7:41 a.m. Medical notes from my nurse indicated that "when the patient was asked about the event, she says that she lost awareness, and she says she just realized that she was in Michigan."

Sixteen minutes later, the nurse said my confusion returned: "She indicates, 'I don't know why I am here.'"

During two confirmed seizures the following day, the nurse wrote that I was sitting down and let out several piercing screams.

"A pedaling motion of the legs is noted while the patient is seated. . . . Just prior to the end of the event, the patient is saying in various tones of voice, 'no, no,' and the intonation of her voice changes."

About fifteen seconds later I was back to reality.

"The patient is answering the examiner's questions appropriately. . . . The patient becomes somewhat, and this is in relative terms, silent and sedated as if she is much calmer."

I took that to mean I was acting normal again and, relative to the screaming, much calmer. At the hospital I recovered from the seizures quickly. That wasn't always the case elsewhere.

Dr. Smith described many of my seizures as "unique" because I talked using random words in various tones at the beginning and the end of the episodes he captured, I wasn't aware I had the events, and I returned to baseline very quickly. "Bizarre" references my strange behaviors—piercing screams, pedaling motion with my legs, and thrashing of my arms and legs, among other things.

"Bizarre" and "unique." Not exactly encouraging words to hear from a neurologist, but I couldn't argue with *bizarre*. How else do you describe a twenty-eight-year-old's tantrum-like seizures in a way that isn't insulting? Reading this in my medical notes now honestly makes me laugh. It's also comforting to know that other neurologists use "bizarre" to explain my types of seizures. Research in the journal *Neurology*, published by the American Academy of Neurology, states that frontal lobe seizures may exhibit bizarre behaviors like thrashing, kicking, unusual facial expressions, and articulate vocalizations.

At that time, the EEG couldn't locate where my seizures were firing from, but Dr. Smith did see activity in the frontal lobe.

Another episode that week started with confusion but quickly spread and created a full-blown seizure.

Dr. Smith first offered to show me a video of the seizure during an appointment following the August 2013 testing. After some hesitation, I convinced myself that watching one of my seizures was important if I was going to understand my epilepsy.

"Are you sure?" he asked.

I nodded, so he pressed play. Up came the video, and within seconds my hands went up in the air, and I let a scream out.

I turned away, mortified. "Uh, stop it. Please stop."

He immediately did. The moment replayed in my head, and I sat down, traumatized. The one nice thing about seizures is that I forgot the bad memories along with the good, so I couldn't recall the few seconds of video I watched that day. Reading my medical notes today, the image of me yelling loudly enough for an entire epilepsy unit to hear crushes me. Those poor nurses, doctors, other patients, their families.

Thankfully my family hasn't had to see this.

My EEG showed spiking over my frontal lobe when I was thrashing my arms and screaming. Frontal lobe seizures have been shown to produce explosive screams and behavior that can appear to be related to a psychiatric disorder, according to the Mayo Clinic. Contrary to what some of its physical symptoms might suggest, epilepsy is not a mental illness; epileptic seizures are short bursts of electrical activity that create chaos in the brain, until everything settles down and the brain returns to baseline.

Six days of seizures went about as well as they could go. Nothing else awry in my body was discovered this time around. But doctors didn't discover where the seizures were starting—called the "onset"—nor could they determine the complete path the seizures were taking. The news was so disappointing. My seizures had returned in full force in 2010, and now, three years later, I still didn't have answers. One reason: all my arm waving and head and neck motions while yelling were contaminating the EEG recording. My movements were creating muscle artifacts, which is muscle activity near the head. All of this made it difficult for Dr. Smith and his team to discern true epileptic activity from muscle artifacts.

Maybe it was frontal lobe epilepsy, but Dr. Smith said other EEG data showed it could be extratemporal lobe epilepsy, meaning the seizures could be starting anywhere but the temporal lobe. Both EEG results would contradict what Dr. Kiley in Oregon had gathered from his testing. Taking everything into account, Dr. Smith diagnosed me with bizarre complex partial seizures that started in one spot but sometimes spread across the entire brain, which are secondary generalization seizures. The EEG just couldn't locate their source.

Though disappointed, I was thankful the seizures had impaired my consciousness, making me unaware of how upset I was. Living

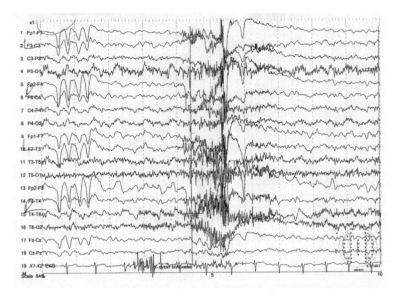

An EEG recording from August 2013 shows my brain waves interrupted by a screaming event during a seizure.

through the screaming would have been awful. It was also a relief that the EEG caught multiple episodes, confirming there was a medical reason for my strange behavior. Dr. Smith later explained it to me:

"Think about when you want to scream. Let's say you're yelling for a family member who is walking in the wrong direction. Your brain has certain areas that control vocalizations, and if those same circuits that control some of those activities are being short circuited or activated by a seizure, that's going to create similar behavior."

A matter-of-fact explanation from an epileptologist was exactly what I needed. It's so incredible how a seizure can completely change someone's behavior within a few seconds, but then the person calms down a short while later as the brain returns to normal. I had never suffered from any physical or emotional trauma, any psychological or psychiatric conditions, so what made me yell "no, no, no!" before starting a screaming rant? My college roommate

Christine said I yelled the same thing during my first seizure in our apartment.

If only there was an easy answer for that one.

Dr. Smith and his colleagues determined that another round of testing in the epilepsy unit would be best and that I could do a presurgical workup there as well. Surgery hadn't entered my mind yet. I was convinced more medication would stop the seizures.

For the time being, they adjusted my medications and sent me on my way. Dr. Smith sent an email to my boss, Ann, the station's general manager, telling her I wasn't allowed to drive for the next six months. Since my seizures had only been happening on my days off—after a long workweek—I had been driving to work and to news stories. Legally, I shouldn't have been driving, but I didn't want to become a burden at work if I wasn't having seizures. His cover letter noted he was a neurologist, but in accordance with the Americans with Disabilities Act (ADA), he didn't need to explain why I couldn't drive.

Ann moved me to the night shift, from 2:30 p.m. to 11:30 p.m., so I could work with Chad, a videographer. I'm a night owl and have a lot of energy in the evening, so I loved the new shift. Chad was easygoing and a hard worker; we made a good team. The seizures stayed at bay, and I was feeling more hopeful each day that the increased medication would work.

But getting to work was a challenge. My walk from home to the office was only a mile, but unlike the smooth bike trails in Eugene, this route was dangerous and full of obstacles. My apartment was tucked back into a quiet, tree-filled neighborhood, but once I walked out the front door, my path to work took me past bustling stores and restaurants, then smack-dab into Interstate 96. To get to work, I'd have to cross the busy on/off ramp over the interstate. My friend and coworker Sarah lived in the same apartment complex, but she worked a different shift, so I couldn't get a ride with her. I rode the city bus occasionally, but it only ran every half hour in the afternoon and stopped running before my shift was over.

So, to get to work on time, running was the fastest method, and it felt safer than biking. The overpass didn't have a sidewalk, so the quicker I crossed it the better. Dodging speedy drivers was terrifying at first, but I soon got used to the areas of my path that required more caution. This was August and September, the perfect temperature for exercising outside. But the winter weather in Grand Rapids isn't mild like in Eugene. Fall turned into winter, creating the perfect slippery conditions for falling flat on my face. Heavy snow boots replaced my light running shoes.

If I missed the bus by a hair, I was punished by walking in freezing rain and snow. Sleet whipped across my face as I trudged carefully over the icy bridge. With no trees to block the harsh, cold wind, I buried my face into my scarf, eyes squinting to spot cars on the days with limited visibility. My body yearned to sprint out of the cold, but I needed to walk to avoid sliding into a vehicle. Exasperation filled drivers' faces as they rolled past, all safe and cozy warm in their vehicles. I could hear their annoyance cut through the wind in the way they lifted a hand off the steering wheel, pointed it toward me, and glared as if to say, "What the hell are you doing? You want to get killed??"

I wanted to shout back, but meeting their gaze would ruin my day, so my eyes stayed glued to the road as I dodged black ice. My winter commute in Eugene felt like a walk in the park compared to this snowy, mile-long trek.

Then there were days when no matter the weather, I would catch the eye of someone who also didn't want to be in harm's way but had no other option. I'd sometimes encounter panhandlers, and occasionally we would nod and acknowledge each other as I walked by. It was easy to brush them off, but my perspective changed when I saw one of their handheld signs up close. A man was holding a sign asking for a small donation to pay for his insulin. What if he had lost his job because of a medical condition and didn't have insurance? In those moments, braving the cold on foot during a dangerous trek to work, I couldn't help but think of how lucky I was to have a job, not to mention insurance.

At the same time, I didn't stop to consider how vulnerable epilepsy had made me on that overpass. A seizure could have struck at any moment, causing a car to seriously injure or kill me. If only I had the confidence then to call the station and ask for a ride, I know someone would have come. But I feared the accommodation would make me appear weak and be one more burden on someone else.

When Chad found out about my commute, he started picking me up and dropping me off after our shifts. His small act of kindness made a huge impact on my ability to get to and from work. Other times, compassion showed up in unexpected places, sometimes from a complete stranger. When a good high school friend was getting married in my hometown, I bought a ticket from Grand Rapids to Minneapolis for a Thursday flight, with the intention of getting a ride home from Minneapolis on Friday. But my brain had other plans.

My flight had a layover in Chicago. Worn out from the workweek, I took a seat at my gate. I don't remember the next part well, just that I had a seizure and a nice man sitting near me happened to be a doctor and recognized the strange behavior. Coming back to awareness following a seizure is alarming enough, but the feeling is amplified in a loud, crowded airport. It was reassuring to have a doctor sitting next to me. I answered his questions, explained that I typically had only one big episode at a time, and said that I would be fine to fly home that night, which I believed was true.

But the public perception of epilepsy is still sadly misunderstood. The gate attendants were frightened by what they saw, so the doctor went up to tell them that I had experienced a seizure but was doing much better and felt fine to fly. With the explanation coming from a doctor, they agreed to let me board. I thanked him profusely, walked onto the plane, and settled into my seat. The flight was almost ready to take off when it happened again. With no warning, a seizure took control of my body, but this time the flight attendants were less understanding. They removed me from the plane and had me transported by ambulance to a hospital six miles away.

The trip to the hospital upset me, not just because I wouldn't get to Minneapolis that night but also because it wasn't necessary. In most cases, seizures are not considered an emergency unless they last for more than five minutes. Mine generally last less than a minute. A doctor evaluated me, determined I was fine, and discharged me around midnight. Exhausted and bleary-eyed, I found a hotel close to the airport where I could crash, grabbed a taxi there, and then scanned flights for the following morning. I fell asleep quickly, not yet aware that the ten-minute ambulance ride and hospital bills would add up to about $3,500. All for a small seizure.

I awoke the next morning to catch my flight, made it through seizure free, and met my mom at the airport to drive north for the wedding. I had kept her informed throughout the ordeal. After meeting Dr. Smith, I was more open with family and friends back home about my disease, though not with anyone at work. Like anyone with epilepsy, I was hopeful, really hopeful, the seizures would stop right away under a new care plan. But they didn't. So I did what I had promised my parents in Oregon and kept them updated.

My mom reminded me that I seemed to understand how worried they were, and I had promised to be more truthful about my seizures. That was a turning point. "Unfortunately, small ones started happening again," I wrote to her. "My brain can handle less sleep than it could in Oregon, but I've learned that if I go more than three days with less than six hours I'm almost guaranteed to have one. I need to catch up on weekends which is why I can easily sleep twelve hours Friday night and ten to twelve hours Saturday night. No grand mals or falls. I'll ask if my meds need to be adjusted again. They always happen at the end of the day."

It was mid-September 2013 by now, three weeks into college football season. As a dedicated Minnesota alumna, I followed the Gophers, but even more so after head coach Jerry Kill revealed he had epilepsy. During one nonconference game against Western Illinois, I read a few updates online and then went on with my day with the intent of looking back later for the final score. A few hours later, the story I was expecting to see was replaced with one that made me gasp. The photo I glanced down at wasn't one of celebration. The Gopher players were all on one knee, their arms linked together, helmets placed by their feet. Solemn expressions filled their sweat-streaked faces, and one player's head was bowed. A police officer blocked the camera's view of what they all gazed down upon.

The big, bold headline provided the answer:

"Jerry Kill suffers another seizure, carted off field."

My eyes welled. Jerry had become an inspiration to me and others as he fought to succeed at a high-profile, demanding job. And now this. A follow-up article noted that he was recovering fine, but my stomach clenched in anticipation of the aftermath—of what sports anchors and columnists would say and write. Of what would fill the comments sections at the bottom of their stories. As a reporter, I was always interested in what viewers and readers had to say, and I usually read both newspaper and Facebook reactions to articles.

The headline stuck with me the rest of the day, so I cut myself off from further media that night. The reaction I feared from the media two days later was even worse than I could have imagined.

"In category of health, Kill falls too short to continue."

I sat back in my chair, folded my arms, and just stared at the headline for a few seconds. Those words carried weight because they came from a longtime Minneapolis sports columnist at the state's largest newspaper, the *Star Tribune*. My hand was already sweating when it clicked the mouse.

"The University of Minnesota's football program, and by extension the entire school, became the subject of pity and ridicule," wrote the columnist. "No one who buys a ticket to TCF Bank Stadium should be rewarded with the sight of a middle-aged man writhing on the ground. This is not how you compete for sought-after players and entertainment dollars."

How could I even react to words so hurtful and ignorant? Half the assumptions made should only come from his doctor. No one else has authority to make such statements. Later that day, after a few thousand angry emails from readers in protest to his article, the columnist wrote, among other things:

"No, I don't think I'm being cruel, I think many of you are being cruel. Kill has had four seizures on game days in 16 home games at Minnesota. The stress of the job seems to have a negative effect on him. You shouldn't want him to put himself in that position for your entertainment."

So now it was readers' fault for defending the football coach? Unbelievable. I wish he could have understood what it was like for someone with epilepsy to read the words "No one . . . should be rewarded with the sight of a middle-aged man writhing on the ground." Jerry Kill is a human being whose medicine didn't control his seizures. Would a columnist be as critical if a person had dropped to the ground due to another medical condition?

I did my best to push away the anger and dismay, but it reinforced my belief that I had to keep my epilepsy a secret. And for a couple months that fall I could, because my seizures were back under control.

But the most maddening part of epilepsy is losing control right when you think you finally have it back. It's like being on the sidelines for months while rehabbing a sports injury, only to get re-injured once you finally get the sweet taste of victory—simply by competing again.

On a warm, late summer afternoon while I was out on a run, my luck ran out. As a result, after roughly four years of living in a state of denial, convincing myself that my seizures were not a problem, I finally took out the seizure journal I had stashed away in a closet. It was blank, just like my memory of almost every seizure. But black ink would soon cover the pages. My denial was over; video EEG had clearly shown something "bizarre, unique, and unusual" going on in my brain, as Dr. Smith had written in my medical chart. So finally, with full acceptance of my disease, it was my job to write down as many details as I could remember.

"I was only planning to run 6 miles so I could pick up my new medication at the Target pharmacy," I wrote in a June 2013 entry. "I ended up running 13 to 14. Somewhere around mile three I lost consciousness [impaired awareness]. No idea where I ran or how I got there, but I made it back to my apartment fine at 12.36 miles. So, I ran longer. I was soaked because it started raining, and I didn't even notice. I was obviously not conscious [my awareness was impaired] because I let my phone get wet, and the speaker didn't work the rest of the night. This has never happened to me before."

Then came a seizure eerily similar to the one that struck on the

Amazon Trail in Oregon. Too similar to forget, it didn't need to go down on paper.

On that day, my legs felt strong as I pushed up a small hill in Grand Rapids on a cold morning in my stocking hat and black leggings. It must have been fall or early winter on a weekend; I was dodging cracks on the sidewalk, parallel to a busy street, when the cars and trees slowly started to blur from the corners of my eyes. Then the incline directly in front of me seemed to magically flatten. My feet turned weightless as my arms propelled me forward into a landscape fading by the second, like rain falling so hard the windshield wipers could no longer clear the road ahead. My brain had entered neverland.

Cars zoomed by, but their engines sounded distant. Then silence. The next memory I have is of standing on a curb, holding onto the metal post of a white traffic sign, with trees and cars coming back into range. My stomach started to sink, my breath falling with it. I gazed down at my legs and feet, then took a long slow look up at the peak of the hill and back down.

How the hell had I run from there to here in a straight line without falling or wading into traffic? Had I passed by anyone?

This was a focal impaired awareness seizure. Though I couldn't recall what had just happened, my brain retained just enough awareness during the seizure to protect me from falling down. It's as if autopilot had turned on. One part of my brain was short-circuiting while the rest of it was directing my body to dodge curbs, trees, people, and cars.

Amazed and frightened, I dropped my hold on the sign and walked the twenty minutes home, on high alert for any strange feelings. My brain stayed calm the rest of the day. Getting lost in my own mind at work was my biggest fear, so I didn't tell anyone about the strange seizures. But I could only hide them for so long.

13

Nowhere Else to Hide

Thankfully, seizures steered clear of the glare of my TV newsroom, mostly happening on weekends. I dodged the bullet at work for more than two years. Hundreds of video shoots, interviews, and live shots were never interrupted by my brain going haywire. But then in February 2014, my luck ran out. I had two seizures at work about three weeks apart. Alana recalls one of them. I came in to work over the weekend, on my day off, to finish up a big story to air the following week. Later that afternoon, Alana was in the weather center preparing the forecast when the seizure struck.

"I could hear your screams in the hallway," she remembered. "I placed my hand on your back and you looked at me straight in the eyes all while crying out loudly (the sound you made sounded like a siren or a fire alarm) until your face turned different shades of blue and purple. I'm not sure how long it lasted. Maybe it was a few minutes, but eventually you stopped and regained the ability to speak and started to ask questions: 'What day is it? Where am I? Why am I here?' You asked the same questions about three times each before you started to fully regain consciousness. I tried to convince you that you needed to go home and rest but you stubbornly insisted that you were okay and that you had to finish your work."

Eventually, I agreed to go home.

Humiliation soon replaced the confusion, once I realized coworkers had just seen what I had tried so hard to hide for so long.

I asked Dr. Smith to talk with my boss, Ann, over the phone. He explained epilepsy and described the type of seizures I had. Ann was proactive in helping educate the staff by drafting a seizure action plan with me. Just three days before she sent it out, one of my coworkers wrote to Ann in confidence about the second seizure

I had experienced at the station. It's the perfect example of why I didn't want to share my epilepsy with anyone.

"I understand that you are aware of the situation and that measures are in place to handle it," the colleague began. "I also want to let you know how much this stresses out the crews that are here at the time when it happens. It interferes with workload and concentration."

There is never a convenient time or place to have a seizure. Whether it's in a newsroom or in thousands of other places, people have seizures every day—in schools and meetings, at gyms and grocery stores, during concerts and sporting events, on airplanes and buses. And while a thirty-second seizure might alarm those who observe it, it's nothing compared to actually having one. Seizures are mentally and physically exhausting, but the worst part for me was finding out people had witnessed them.

Ann sent out an email to the entire staff with the finalized seizure action plan. A few coworkers were willing to be emergency responders, which I was so grateful for.

"In the event that a seizure does happen in the workplace, it is wise to be prepared," the plan stated. "A properly implemented plan of action may reduce the confusion, panic, or fear that coworkers or customers experience if they see an employee having a seizure on the job."

The plan went on to describe warning signs and to outline actions to be taken.

"The station emergency responder provides first aid and stays with Stacia until she recovers. The station emergency responder also makes the decision on whether we need to call 911. The highest ranking manager on duty in the newsroom calls Stacia's mom or dad. If there is no manager on duty, then the emergency responder should direct someone else in the station to make the call. Stacia's contact phone numbers are posted at her desk."

It went on to give first aid assistance information and guidelines of what not to do, including placing anything in my mouth or restraining me during a seizure. I read through the entire email, then let out the breath I seemed to have been holding for months.

Would anyone reply?

The silence made me nervous. I had already sensed that some people were irritated with me, but would there be any empathy?

A message from Chad soon appeared in my inbox with an un-expected response: "I know that it's a rough situation for you to be in, Stacia. You are a strong woman and I know that it can be tough to acknowledge what others might perceive as a weakness. But every one of us here and in the larger world has issues that we struggle with, and they only become more difficult if we refuse to recognize them and don't accept help from our friends and teammates. I'm glad that your struggle has been outed, because it makes the problem a challenge to face and cope with rather than a source of cruel or ignorant gossip. I for one am happy to drive you wherever you need to go, both for work and to and from your home. You live too close to work for that to be an issue. No more busing in the middle of the night during the dead of winter for you! I enjoy your company and I'm happy to chase stories with you all over Michigan."

Chad copied Ann in his reply. His support was a total surprise and meant the world to me at the time. He gave me confidence to walk back into the newsroom, and six years later, his letter still pops into my thoughts occasionally, sometimes making me smile, other times making me tear up. Chad was the first person to ac-knowledge why I felt the way I did and why I shouldn't have to feel that way. He was also the first person to help me grasp that other people also struggle to hide their own insecurities. I contacted him while writing this book, to ask about what he remembered from that time. We had worked together often, and his answer shocked me. What I thought was a "small seizure" right before a live shot at Michigan State University had been anything but small.

In April 2014, the Spartans men's basketball team, coach Tom Izzo, and hundreds of students were holding a vigil for a little girl who had died of cancer. Princess Lacey, as she was called, and one of the team's players, Adreian Payne, had formed a close bond after he visited her in the hospital. Players and students took turns writing their condolences on a large rock on the East Lansing campus. Media from across Michigan showed up, and TV reporters, including myself, were doing last-minute mic checks before we went live. We all spread out to find quiet spots, and for that I am grateful.

Chad shared his memory from that night with me because I don't have one:

> We were just a couple minutes away from going live, and I
> saw you kind of zone out for a second. I asked if you were okay
> a few times, and then you suddenly came to and let out a blood
> curdling shriek. I can still hear it in my mind, I had never
> heard a sound like that before. Of all the scary things folks like
> us see in news, that one really stuck with me. Then you gave
> me a terrified look, like you thought I was attacking you and
> you were trying to get away from me, even though it was kind
> of the other way around. That lasted maybe a few seconds,
> then you were quickly back to normal. I had no idea what
> had just happened, but I called the executive producer and
> told them to cut away. Right after that you were really sad and
> upset that you had missed the live shot, and you insisted on
> going into the event to try and get video and some interviews.
> I tried to get you to relax for a minute but you were adamant.
> I couldn't go after you because I had all the camera gear and
> live equipment set up. In hindsight knowing what I know now
> I feel really bad that I let you just wander off after what had
> happened . . . but I just didn't know what to do at the time.
> Once you came back you seemed totally fine, and I barely
> remember the drive home.

My jaw dropped. Talk about bizarre. The mixed messages flying around my brain that evening had led me to scream and think Chad was attacking me out of the blue, during regular conversation? You can't make this stuff up.

Three years had passed since my last live shot was ruined, back in Oregon in 2010. Once Chad and I got back to the station and I wrote the news story about the vigil, I headed into the audio booth to voice it. The strange, stupid mistake I made in there still baffles me to this day.

My script said "Adreian Payne," but for some strange reason I said "Adrian Smith." The latter is a congressman in Nebraska whose work I had covered six years prior. Looking back, my brain still must have been in the postictal state—recovering from the large seizure. But my state of mind following this seizure alarmed my coworkers. The nightside executive producer informed me I could no longer go live. I was no longer 100 percent dependable. My first reaction was sheer embarrassment. Yes, it was a stupid mistake, but it hadn't been deliberate. Deep down, though, I knew the error was a big one. Viewers were probably left scratching their heads, wondering how a young reporter could screw up the name of a local college basketball star.

Recording a Michigan State basketball player's last name wrong was my only on-air mistake, thankfully, but off-air, my memory problems were starting to show. I didn't know it at the time, but Zonisamide was affecting my memory, concentration, attention, and thinking, and for that reason, I would be taken off of it the following year. I hated not feeling sharp. My stories were taking longer to write as I pleaded with my brain to think of the right words and recall important details.

One of my coworkers told Ann she was concerned about my memory because I'd been forgetting so much over the past six months. I was just as frustrated with myself as some of my colleagues were. Yes, seizures and the medication were the cause. But, ultimately, I was responsible for recalling important information to write my stories by deadline.

As a result, I'd lose sleep over my news stories. More of my weekends were now spent in darkness, with the curtains drawn and a white noise machine turned on for twelve hours each night, hoping to create the right conditions to help me sleep.

The seizures were sporadic; I'd have a few in a row, but then two or three weeks would pass, sometimes longer, with nothing. How could my memory have gotten so bad with only a handful of seizures a month? I never thought to consider whether I was having seizures without knowing it, because at that time, I didn't even know that was possible.

Losing my live shot privileges hurt, but it would have been much harder to walk back into that newsroom if Chad hadn't covered for me. That definitely was no "small seizure." He could have told everyone what really happened, but he chose compassion instead.

"I never told anyone at the station about how it went down because it would be impossible to relay that kind of story to newspeople without sensationalizing it," he told me. I'm hopeful there are more people like Chad in newsrooms, or any workplace, out there.

Eventually I got over the feeling of being a burden at work. Reporting revealed a bigger picture, where my insecurity over someone's perception of me was insignificant compared to real-world problems. In the rush of daily news, sometimes TV reporters get opportunities to do more in-depth pieces, and the personal stories left lasting impressions on me.

In Nebraska, Oregon, and Michigan I interviewed people from every walk of life. Most seemed hesitant to share their hardships at first, like losing their jobs due to massive layoffs or, worse, losing a child to cancer. Earning the trust of strangers was my job, but sometimes I felt myself tear up listening to their experiences. Reporting every day brought constant reminders that someone had it worse than me, even with epilepsy. Seizures had become an inconvenience, I believed, not something pitiable.

At that point, I was still only looking at the day-to-day limitations of my epilepsy, believing my seizures were well enough under control to keep reporting full-time. My glossy outlook kept my perspective in the here and now. Things weren't so bad, I told myself, and my mostly positive attitude helped me convince friends and loved ones that things were fine. I didn't grasp at the time, though, that controlling seizures "well enough" wasn't good enough. If seizures aren't completely controlled, they can worsen over time, and every seizure increases the risk of an accident.

Maybe my determined outlook was attributed to years of playing sports. Sports psychologists have studied how negative thoughts can often lead to negative performance, and I found that to be true in tennis for sure. If I let myself think negatively after a forced error, the rest of the match would often go off in a tailspin. College athletes are constantly bouncing back from injuries and bad races. When I was racing in college, injuries were frustrating, but they trained me to be resilient. When you fall down, you get back up again or you're done. Someone else will take your spot on the team.

In the same way, I had to pick myself up after every awful seizure and go on with my day or I wouldn't have had a career. This is not to say it was easy—AT ALL. Many seizures left me in tears and with feelings of hopelessness in that moment. But I knew that falling into a trap of negativity could spiral into depression.

A few months after the seizure in East Lansing, I boarded a flight to Washington, DC, to see Kara. The Air Force Academy had recently stationed her husband, Ben, there, and they had relocated. Due to my health issues, I hadn't taken a real vacation since moving to Michigan, and I was excited to see the sights. And I was feeling good. But the entire trip exists only in my scrapbook—a seizure erased the vacation from my memory.

"It took me a couple seconds to realize it was happening," Kara recalled.

It was the day we went out to Annapolis, to see the cute shops, the Naval Academy, and take a boat tour of the harbor. We were in our small apartment downtown D.C. relaxing and talking around 10 p.m. During our conversation, you suddenly just seemed to space out. You weren't really responding, and you were seemingly motionless. You were staring off somewhere. Realizing it was a seizure, I calmly kept saying, "Stacia, hey Stacia, you OK?" Once you did begin speaking again, you asked questions in a confused manner. You said you had to go to the bathroom, so you went, then you came back. Only a minute later, you would once again say you had to use the bathroom, and you would go again. You did this about 4 times. About 20 minutes after the seizure, I noticed you were troubled and disturbed. Before I could even tell you that you had had a seizure, you straight out asked me if you had had a seizure. You knew. You then explained that you had forgotten to take your meds that morning, which was likely the cause.

That was the last time I could convince Kara that things were fine, even if I was on a good stretch of seizure freedom. She had never witnessed a seizure until that visit, and, as she recalled, that kept the reality of what I was going through distant for her. Though we didn't avoid mentioning seizures, we never really had an open conversation about epilepsy. Maybe not talking about it gave me unconscious permission to not confront my growing fears.

After we said our goodbyes, I made a quick sightseeing trip to New York City before returning home, upset that Kara had had to witness a seizure but relieved that she now better understood them and only had to see a small one. Witnessing me overtaken by déjà vu or jamais vu would have been much scarier. Those auras are longer and more intense.

14

Jamais Vu

The sun was setting as I sat down to eat dinner at the small living room table in my Michigan apartment. Halfway into my meal, my surroundings gradually started to shift. Looking down at my plate, the food started to look different and pale in color.

Is that chicken on my plate? Is that a stir-fry? Did I make that?

The food instantly became tasteless, so I put my fork down and pushed my plate away. Hospital video EEG had recorded me doing the same thing.

I looked up to see paper bags filled with groceries on the counter.

Why are bags there? Did I go grocery shopping before this? And when? What kind of food did I buy?

The pink salmon peeked out from the corner of one bag.

Gross. Fish? Do I eat fish?

Overwhelmed, my entire body tensed as I scanned the room, carefully studying everything from the rugs to the blanket on my couch to the wicker basket on the shelf.

Where did that blanket come from?

Is this even my place?

Yes, it has to be my place.

Where else would I be?

Fear rose in my chest. *In that moment I knew I was experiencing jamais vu. Everything should have looked familiar, but it was like I was seeing it all for the first time.*

I felt like an intruder in my own apartment. My gaze wandered around the kitchen. The stainless-steel refrigerator and shiny stove looked brand-new.

Have I ever cooked on that before?

Pinkish-red apples peeked out from another paper bag.

Apples . . . apples . . . yes, I eat apples.

The bag was full, but the vibrant assortment of red blurred together, so I shifted my gaze to another wall.

A small piano stood to my right.

Why is that there? Do I play piano?

I gave my brain a couple seconds.

Nothing. I spotted cookbooks on the shelf. *Do I bake?* The thought of chocolate chip cookies fresh out of the oven at that second made me feel nauseous.

Stay in your chair. The seizure might get worse.

I lost awareness for a bit because the next thing I remember is opening my eyes and peeking through my hands. The seizure had passed, but now confusion took over while my brain recovered. Unlike jamais vu—where I was on high alert and knew my surroundings should have looked familiar—the postictal state was brain fog to the extreme.

What time is it? What day is it?

"Where am I?" I whispered, putting my head into my hands and slowly glancing around. The beige walls offered no clues.

Exhaustion overwhelmed me as I leaned back in the chair. My head stayed cradled in my hands, waiting for the confusion to diminish. I sat there for probably around twenty seconds, but it seemed closer to twenty minutes.

The geese honking outside my window turned my attention to the patio, where a few waddled around in search of food.

Wait, geese? Have geese always lived around here?

I stood up and walked to the kitchen to get a look out the window. A few cars drove past, but nothing clicked. Still confused, I glanced back to the countertop and opened the fridge, hoping the details of the interior of my place would help my brain match the exterior. I peered out the window again, but held my gaze this time. Something connected with the green landscape of manicured lawns, trees, plants, and rocks placed around the building.

"Michigan! I am in Michigan and this is where I work! I'm a reporter!" I exclaimed.

But where do I work?

I squeezed my eyes again, begging my brain to wake up. I looked down and saw my purple dress. I was wearing a dress and cute shoes.

Why am I sitting in my apartment dressed up?

Straight ahead a small hallway led toward a room. My bedroom. Still somewhat disoriented, I stood up and made my way to the room, past my bed and nightstand, and opened the two folding doors to my closet and stepped inside. Hopefully clothes would jog my memory. But scanning red, then blue, then black blouses left me clueless. I looked across the room, then out the window, then sighed in defeat and sat down on the floor. After a few moments of silence, the puzzle pieces of my life that were scattered about slowly started to find their place back together.

A TV graphic sprang to mind.

The TV station was close by, close enough to walk.

Wait, did I work today?

I glanced down.

I'm in a dress, so I must have. What did I report on today?

Again, I drew a blank. It was all I could handle for the night. I looked at my phone.

Oh, thank God, it's a Friday. I don't work tomorrow.

I was relieved to recognize my bed just a few feet away. Twelve hours of sleep Friday night would reset my brain and give me a fresh start for the week. This was my routine each weekend. Sleep was my ticket to seizure freedom, and the next morning my body felt 100 percent again.

Wait, what did I do yesterday?

My mind rewound the tape.

Oh, that's right, the seizure. That's why I slept so long.

The day following a seizure was always the "let's see what Stacia remembers" day. I racked my brain for work stories.

Monday and Tuesday . . .

"Crap. What did I do?" I said out loud.

Nothing came up.

Wednesday, I think it was a Wednesday when I covered an unde-tected tornado?

But Thursday and Friday were a blank slate.

Anger set in, knowing that another forgotten week would hurt me in the long run. Running was the only thing that cured frustration, but since it sometimes triggered seizures, staying in was the safest option. Sure, I could have vented to friends or family over the phone instead, but at twenty-nine years old, dumping my feelings on someone else's shoulders felt like whining. Relationships need to be a give-and-take, I believed, and all there was to offer on my end was taking. Most of all, though, nobody knew what the bewildering aftermath of a seizure was like or what living with the challenges of epilepsy entailed, so what could they possibly offer me? Part of me wanted to meet a friend with epilepsy who understood what it felt like to be an outsider. Another part of me wanted to keep everything bottled up and busy myself with distractions. Facebook support groups didn't exist yet, so I didn't know where to turn. My journal? Turning the page to write about yet another seizure wasn't therapeutic—it enraged me.

"Fuck the journal!" I shouted, throwing it angrily into the closet. A pen would never touch those pages again.

Saturday night brought ten more hours of deep sleep. The next morning my body felt great, but walking into the kitchen to see the oven and refrigerator again soured my happy mood. I desperately needed a mental boost, so I tied my shoes, grabbed my Garmin watch and iPod, and jogged down the stairs. My legs would run as far as my body would let them today, I decided, confident that all that sleep would prevent a storm from brewing. And it did. The pace was easy; I didn't bust out of the gate hard but instead just enjoyed the feeling of freedom. There's nothing more freeing than good health. After barely breaking a sweat, I returned home with a smile on my face, grateful to move my body and letting myself believe once again that things would be fine.

The one detail I failed to remember was that each of my seizures had repercussions. The hard-fought reality that my worsening

memory would eventually make reporting impossible if the seizures continued had not completely set in. Epilepsy had already
taken away my personal life and marathon racing, but the possibility of losing my career seemed impossible. I never could have
imagined that a seizure could affect so many other people.

15

Epilepsy Wins

I nearly fell out of my chair when I heard her words. My jaw dropped, and I stopped breathing for a few seconds. I was sitting in front of Ann's large desk in a sprawling office on the second floor of the TV station. My new news director, Richard, looking uneasy, also sat with us. Ann had called me on my day off and asked me to come in, which I thought was strange. It was Thursday, and on Tuesday I had had two seizures at work.

A knot was growing in my stomach. My gut reaction was that some of my reporting privileges would be taken away because of what had happened at the courthouse.

"Do you know what happened on Tuesday?" Ann asked.

The entire day was a blur. The workday started at 9:00 a.m. with a daily news meeting, when the news director and the day-side crew—me, fellow reporters, photographers, and producers— would gather around a long table in the middle of the newsroom. Each morning, our eyes fixed on the news director, who gave a rundown of stories from the previous night's 11:00 p.m. show and that morning's show. Then we got to work on the 5:00 p.m. and 6:00 p.m. broadcasts; reporters and producers pitched story ideas, and we discussed follow-ups to recent stories, press releases from local cities and counties, court cases, school board meetings, non-profit events, ribbon cuttings, and the occasional feature. Some of the best story ideas came from viewers' emails.

That day, July 22, I was sent to the Kent County Courthouse to cover a case. My memory of the entire day is limited to a few split-second flashbacks, but I was later able to piece things together from coworkers' accounts, emails, and testimony in my work file. All of the following dialogue and information comes directly from conversations documented by either my boss or news director, as well as Alana. I don't recall anything from the courthouse.

Shortly after 2:00 p.m., a detective called my TV station to let them know that I was having some type of episode, that I was confused about where I was and why I was there, and that he would stay with me until help arrived. Alana told me that I had texted her because I had felt a seizure coming on. She drove over to the courthouse and found me upstairs in the press conference room, sitting cross-legged on the floor with a water bottle next to the detective and a photographer from our TV station, Jason.

Alana told me I was upset and exhausted but appeared coherent.

Jason led me to the elevator and later told Richard and Ann that I was disoriented and concerned for my job.

"She began to look strange on the elevator ride," he told them, saying that I didn't get off when the doors opened, so we rode it again. When I did get out the second time, he said, I was confused about what was going on.

Once I got back to the station, Ann found me, and we headed for Richard's office. She said I told them I was fine—but clearly I wasn't.

When they asked me where I was, they said I replied:

"We're at his house. Yeah, yeah, we're at his house," while I was nodding at Richard. I had never been to Richard's house, and I didn't even know where he lived.

My brain was still in the postictal state of confusion, which usually stretched from a few seconds to a few hours for me. I didn't remember what had happened in the courtroom or the elevator ride. Later in the conversation, Ann said, I didn't remember making the comment about Richard's house.

Ann and Richard asked me to get a ride home with someone and rest.

Ann left, and Richard said I asked about doing live shots in the future and about a job opening at another station within the company. He replied that we needed to get through the week first. Richard said I also asked what day of the week it was. Date and time are two questions people have told me I have asked on repeat while trying to make sense of the world again following a seizure.

I then left Richard's office, and this is the point where my memory resurfaces for a minute. I remembered my coworker Ashley, who had approached me recently to ask about epilepsy because someone she knew had started having seizures. Now seemed like a good moment to check in, so I stepped into her office.

Two hours had passed since my courthouse seizure, and I had failed to consider that my brain could easily generate another seizure at any time. I also didn't know that it was possible for strange behavior to occur during the postictal state without having any awareness or memory of doing it. Without an EEG it was impossible to know, but one of the two explains what happened next in her office.

I don't remember what I said or how long I was in there—but the last thing I saw was a split-second shot of another coworker showing me something at an edit bay. Then lights out.

My entire mind went black in a second.

In my brain on that day, either a seizure or a prolonged postictal state left me physically and cognitively unable to keep from being swept up in a new wave of the destruction.

In the aftermath, my next memory was of waking up confused on a couch in the green room with Ashley and Alana, who were comforting me. They insisted that I go home to rest. No one told me what had happened in Ashley's office, so I assumed I had had an embarrassing yelling fit and finally agreed to leave. Alana drove me home and walked me upstairs to my apartment to make sure I was OK. The directions in the seizure action plan were not followed by anyone in management that day.

Neither my mom nor my dad received a phone call, and my work file shows no one even attempted to call them. Nor does it show that anyone called 911. The plan explicitly instructs someone to call 911 if the seizure stops and is followed by another seizure without the person fully regaining consciousness.

This is a gray area—in reviewing the detailed notes from

management in my work file, it appears that I had a seizure at the courthouse, went through a long postictal state afterward, and was still confused when I left Richard's office. I definitely wasn't back to 100 percent if I was asking what day of the week it was.

Once I reached my colleague's office, it's impossible to know if my postictal state stretched even further, which would have been unusually long for me, or if I had a second seizure. My work file says I had a third seizure on the couch in the green room, before Alana drove me home. I had another seizure at some point that evening.

Multiple seizures over the course of a few hours is referred to as a seizure cluster. Clusters can be dangerous because there's a higher chance the seizures will evolve into status epilepticus—a prolonged seizure that can cause death.

According to the seizure action plan, management had not been in the wrong for not calling 911. I had regained consciousness after the courthouse seizure, though I definitely wasn't back to normal. But why didn't my boss and news director, who both witnessed my confusion during our conversation, follow the protocol and call my parents in Minnesota? Instead, they offered a ride home. My brain clearly wasn't recovering, so the next step should have been the hospital to get evaluated and monitored. Looking back, if my parents had been called, they would have insisted on it.

As my head hit the pillow quickly that Tuesday night, my thoughts were swimming.

What had happened? Was it worse than the other seizures I'd had earlier that year at work?

The questions ran through my mind as I fell in and out of sleep. I had the following two days off, Wednesday and Thursday, for which I was grateful. Two days off would reset my brain. But on Thursday afternoon, Ann called.

"Stacia, can you come to my office today, please?"

Her tone made me nervous.

I wondered why she needed to talk with me today, why it couldn't wait until tomorrow.

I slid my shoes on for the walk to work, my mind racing. Once

I arrived and knocked on the door to her office, both Ann and Richard greeted me with grim expressions and motioned for me to take a seat.

Ann then proceeded to tell me something else that apparently happened, which, to this day, is impossible for me to comprehend. My behavior in my colleague's office had escalated to cause something far worse than waving my arms around and screaming. I'll never forget the emotions that boiled over.

Ann said I had acted out toward my colleague in an inappropriate way.

Then words came flying out of my mouth in short, defensive gasps.

"Oh my God. Are you joking? That's never happened before."

I was crying now.

People had witnessed my seizures in the past—at the airport, in the newsroom, even during TV interviews—but I had never actually touched another person during a seizure. The closest thing I had done was turn around and stare at a coworker, not aware I was doing so. This couldn't be real.

"I have to ask my doctor if he's seen that before," I said.

Ann told me I was suspended with pay until Monday, and then we would meet to discuss the next steps.

"We'll talk on Monday about your future," she said, saying the incident needed to be investigated first.

"Will you talk to my doctor right now?" I begged, desperate for her to realize I wasn't the awful person I had just been made out to be.

I wanted to crawl into a corner and hide from the world. But first I had to get out of her office, and as quickly as possible.

Tears clouded my vision as I stepped outside and opened my phone in a quick search for my hospital's number. The clock was ticking. It was already after four o'clock, and I knew my chance of reaching Dr. Smith was minimal at best, but I had never wanted someone to answer the phone so badly in my life. His nurse answered, she put me on hold, and he took my call. What he said to Ann both relieved and devastated me.

Dr. Smith explained that though I did not knowingly put a hand on my coworker, it is possible for someone to do that during a seizure.

"Behavior in the brain is a balance type of phenomenon. So when you don't have the full system in line, it can create or result in activity you don't want to do," he said.

Dr. Bertram told me that it's very difficult to say what the source of certain behaviors is during seizures, because it's related more to how a seizure spreads, not where it starts. At that time, we didn't know where my seizures were starting from. In some cases, he says, the more obvious seizure-related behaviors are actually postictal and occur while the brain returns to baseline.

"I have a few patients who become very affectionate after a seizure and will hug almost anything," he told me. "One time it happened to be a hot wood stove. She got third-degree burns as a result. Some patients become aggressive after the seizure, not during. We have no idea why."

Dr. Arthur Cukiert, professor of neurosurgery at the University of Sao Paulo and head of the Epilepsy Surgery Program at Clinica Cukiert in Sao Paulo, Brazil, echoed Dr. Bertram. He told me that inappropriate behavior can be seen during a seizure but that the behavior has also been seen after many types of seizures.

"You might have had either a prolonged postictal confusion or a second seizure that added a second postictal state."

If it wasn't a seizure, he confirmed why I didn't remember anything after I blacked out in Ashley's office.

"It is quite common for people not to recall at all what happened during the confusional postictal state," he added. "It is non-voluntary."

I left immediately after Ann and Dr. Smith ended their call, went home, and collapsed on the couch in a bundle of disbelief and tears. What had happened? This was my fifth year of living with epilepsy. I finally felt like I was making progress, and then this—the single worst day of seizures I'd ever had in my life. At least the wave of seizures following the marathon in Seattle had taken place in my apartment, so I had avoided the added pain of witnesses and humiliation. The cuts and bruises that weekend in no way compared to this.

Over the last four months I had brought my epilepsy more under control. I still experienced a few breakthrough seizures, but I truly felt I was on my way to complete control with my medications. My upward climb came crashing down on that July afternoon. I hadn't slept well Sunday night, and on that Tuesday, my brain simply betrayed me.

16

Termination

I wouldn't need to wait until the following Monday for a response from the station. Ann called me back into work the next day, Friday morning. This part I remember. The meeting, documented by the news director, was brief.

"We are terminating you effective immediately," she said in a serious tone, with an expression to match.

I gasped. Before the words could register, she started to read my termination letter aloud.

"Dear Stacia: This letter is to confirm that your last day of employment is today. The reason for this action is your conduct . . ."

"Your conduct."

My ears clung to those two words, and I stopped listening. Then my brain started to rewind:

"Your."

Meaning me.

Stacia.

No, no, no. This couldn't be happening. This was a nightmare.

I truly did think the information from Dr. Smith would change her mind.

"Did my doctor's comments not weigh in at all?"

"The reason for it doesn't matter," she replied coolly. "We can't condone it."

Tears fell quickly, a hot mix of anger and humiliation.

"Someone with a medical condition—you fire them like that. I've worked my butt off since I have been here. You don't care."

"You know we have been accommodating. This has escalated to a different level."

How could I make sense of a letter that said I touched someone after I blacked out? I'd never interacted with anyone during a seizure or in the postictal state before. My intention was simply to check in on the person with epilepsy my coworker knew.

I had no way of knowing what was accurate regarding my actions. I really didn't even want to know. One thing I did know is that I would *never* consciously lay a hand on someone. But how could I defend myself when I had no recollection of what truly happened that day?

"I can't look at myself in the mirror. I'm so ashamed. I would never do that. I couldn't sleep last night," I told Ann.

She told me to turn in my station cell phone and laptop on Monday.

I wiped away my tears, stood up, left her office, and headed into the newsroom with my head down, my eyes focused on the ground. I grabbed the various belongings still on my desk and left the station. My short walk home was like walking along the shore of nearby Lake Michigan. Each footprint was immediately washed away. Never again would my feet walk that path to and from the station, or possibly any station. Remembering my promise to keep my parents informed, I took out my phone and called my mom as I walked.

"Hello, Stacia!" she said after a few rings.

"They fired me" is all I could manage to say back. My mom heard every emotion I was feeling in those three words. Disbelief, anger, and sadness.

"What?! Why?! When should I catch a plane to Grand Rapids to be with you?" Her words came out in a rush.

"Wait, wait," I said, trying to calm her down. "You don't need to come out right away. I just . . . don't . . . know . . . what to do. What am I supposed to do? Look for a new job here? I need a job. What about my health insurance? What about . . ."

My pulse quickened.

"What about my medications?! Are they still covered? Can I still call my doctor?"

My inner voice stopped me.

Stop panicking! There isn't time. One thing at a time. What's the most pressing thing right now? Your health. Call Dr. Smith.

We hung up once I reached my apartment. My mom couldn't believe how quickly I had switched from disbelief, anger, and tears to determination to take action. Moving quickly felt like my only option. My head was swimming with the number of people I needed to call in the next few hours before everything closed for the weekend—my doctor, pharmacy, and insurance company. But once I stepped into my apartment, I broke down as tears blanketed my cheeks.

"It was epilepsy, not me!" I yelled, walking through the entryway to my living room. "I didn't choose to do that! I wasn't even conscious! I would never, ever, ever hurt someone! Never!"

I dropped to the couch, crushed under the weight of my emotions, and lay there motionless for a good ten minutes, trying to comprehend how my world could have fallen apart so unexpectedly. Then I looked at the clock. Time to pick up the phone.

"Keep it together. You can't cry to people on the phone," I coached myself.

Just as I was starting to make calls, my mom was answering a call from a Grand Rapids, Michigan, area code. She had a feeling she knew who it was.

"I am concerned about Stacia and wanted to make sure you are in contact with her," Ann told my mom.

"I'm aware of what's going on. My husband and I have to decide whether to go now or wait until she's ready to pack up. I'm sorry it happened," my mom replied.

"I can't go into any details, but I just want to make sure that Stacia had contacted you," Ann said.

The call was unknown to me until I saw it later in my work file. I shook my head in disbelief.

" 'Concerned'? Are you kidding me?"

Not all my questions were answered from the work file when I started writing this book, so I turned to Alana for help. She told me she was shocked when she found out I had been fired.

"No one told me anything about what had happened," she said. "I was so hurt for you and angry. I called Ashley and asked what had happened and why no one had talked to me since I picked you up from the courthouse and took you home from the station that day."

Alana said Ashley answered the call in tears. "She said that she filed a complaint with the hope that it would lead to a medical leave of absence and a chance for you to get the medical attention you needed without having to worry about work."

This was all news to me. My view softened a little because a medical leave of absence is what I had been hoping for in the days following the incident.

Meanwhile, in my apartment, after my last "Thank you for your help," I hit the red button on my phone to end the call and burst into tears. Some good news was that I could still get my medications, for now. But I still had to process an unfathomable morning.

"Your conduct."

The words in ink didn't need a second glance—they left a permanent impression in my mind. Memory loss could never erase them.

The anger that consumed me all day soon gave way to a stronger emotion.

Hurt.

Anger came in quick bursts, settled down, and then came back again. Once the hurt set in that night, it took hold of my thoughts.

17

The Best Place to Start Over

Before July 22, 2014, my career had clarity. But when the neurons in my brain short-circuited that day, that clarity disappeared as quickly as switching off a light. What would "normal" feel like again? Could I ever be a reporter again? As a journalist, all my stories had a beginning, middle, and end. Every day. Sometimes the ending was wonderful. Other times it was expected, sad, surprising, exciting, or just plain awful. And sometimes the narrative would change overnight, and my job would be to update everything the next day. The story of my own life has a happy beginning; the middle had been a mix of ups and downs, similar to other people's experiences before the age of thirty. But through it all, I was still getting up every morning and plugging away.

That is, until July 22, when the biggest storm of my life tore across my brain and quickly left its mark. In its wake, a horrible truth made itself known.

I could no longer trust my own brain.

I couldn't trust it to make normal, appropriate decisions. That day, my brain failed to protect me. It had been failing me for some time. It had failed to remember things big and small, from important conversations to a bridesmaid's dress at an airport. Brainstorms had sent my mind (and body) wandering astray on my favorite trail only two blocks from my house. They had frightened loved ones across the country, like Sara in her San Francisco apartment, Kara in her Washington, DC, apartment, and my parents in a Grand Rapids hospital. Brainstorms had targeted me physically—breaking a tooth, cutting my eye on a desk during a fall, and slicing my arm with a knife. Brainstorms had taken away some of the best moments of my life.

And now a brainstorm had brought an abrupt end to my reporting career.

That moment forced me to finally face my disease head-on. Hoping that more medication would solve my problems while I considered new tests would simply be another detour. My journey had hit a dead end. Hope needs action at some point, and I had spent a very long decade trying to run away from epilepsy, trusting that more medication and sleep would solve it.

Sometimes rock bottom is the best place to start over.

Don't give up on yourself, Stacia.

Glossing over the frustration helped me avoid worrying others. But I had ended up hurting family and friends along the way, and now a coworker. The next two weeks in Grand Rapids went by in a mix of disbelief, stress, and determination that played out like a never-ending tennis match. An internal Q and A kept me bouncing back and forth.

Had my TV station violated the ADA?

Find an attorney.

How can I afford rent without a job? And food? And health insurance?

Find a new job.

Can I ever be a reporter again?

Move back to Minnesota.

If I moved back to my home state, would I find a new doctor or stay with Dr. Smith and fly back for treatment?

No, use your head—that's too expensive. Find a new epileptologist in the Twin Cities.

Trying to answer those questions humbled me. When everything is going right in life, it's easy to tell someone to "just get a new job." But as with other chronic diseases, it's not that easy to do with epilepsy. A life with epilepsy requires a job that offers sick leave and good health insurance to cover appointments, imaging, neuropsychology tests, medications, a week of inpatient video EEG testing, follow-up visits, and possibly implants or brain surgery with a long recovery period.

Nor is it easy to get a new job when your medical condition is stigmatized, you've been terminated unexpectedly, and you don't know the barriers you're facing. With so many phone calls to make and emails to send in so little time, there was no time for self-pity.

Out of everything on my to-do list, my most important task was to find a doctor. The last thing I wanted was to start all over with someone new, but for financial, practical, and emotional reasons, to truly move on, I needed to move back to Minnesota.

To move forward with my health, I needed insurance.

But what kind of health insurance could I get without a job lined up? And would it cover epilepsy care?

Plopping down onto my couch, I scoured Google to research my options.

I keyed in "How to get health insurance if you don't have a job."

MNsure and Medical Assistance popped up.

I had heard of MNsure. Just a year earlier, in 2013, Minnesota had established the Minnesota Insurance Marketplace to help people purchase individual plans if they didn't have one through an employer.

But Medical Assistance was foreign to me.

It was Minnesota's Medicaid program, health insurance coverage for those who didn't make enough money to pay basic living expenses, let alone medical bills. Based on their requirements, I would qualify. I just needed to fill out the paperwork.

I fell back onto the couch in shock.

After paying the maximum out-of-pocket fees for insurance the last two years—which had eaten up a big chunk of my salary—free healthcare when I needed it most seemed like a godsend.

I'd put my savings toward rent and food while I looked for a job.

With the most important financial lifeline of my life in place, the next step was finding the right epileptologist. Dr. Smith had someone in mind who worked at a clinic in Saint Paul. He trusted she would be the best fit to treat me, and I trusted him. I called the Minnesota Epilepsy Group and asked if Dr. Patricia Penovich was taking new patients. The answer disappointed me. She was booked for at least the next six months. I relayed the information back to Dr. Smith, who called her himself. Suddenly, I was her patient.

After playing the waiting game to get treatment in the past, I was overjoyed at the quick response.

I was set to see Dr. Penovich on October 20, in about three months. I sat down on my couch and let the news sink in. Success number one. For the first time since receiving my termination letter, the uncertainty of my future started to fade. The most important thing during the hardest part of my life was the first thing to go right that week. Getting a new doctor at home, where I had my support system, helped me mentally start seeing a successful path forward.

The next morning, new window browsers on my laptop screen popped up continuously, my fingers typing away as I searched for information on epilepsy surgery, published research to explain my alleged actions, jobs in the Twin Cities, and employment attorneys. The Epilepsy Foundation's Jeanne A. Carpenter Epilepsy Legal Defense Fund popped up in the search bar. I leaned in closer. An entire fund to help people who've lost their jobs to epilepsy. I felt a little less alone. I submitted a description of my situation right away on the website and anxiously awaited a reply. In the meantime, I made more calls and sent out emails to share the news, while also apartment hunting and managing all the things that come with a big move.

I became a hermit in my living room, alternating between sitting at my desk writing emails, pacing around the kitchen, and breaking down on the floor. The sight of the carpet in my living room is ingrained in my mind. When picking myself off the floor and walking to my desk, I'd notice a trail of small, thin balls of hair on the carpet. It took me a few days to realize that stress was causing my hair to fall out. Finding a new job felt daunting, and each day brought the stark realization that staying in my chosen field might not be possible. Losing the career I loved because of something beyond my control destroyed my belief that hard work always pays off in the end. It had paid off in marathon training and in moving from one TV station to the next. But hard work didn't matter this time. Epilepsy had won.

The two things picking me up off the floor each day were the nonstop support from my amazing network of family and friends and the reassurance from Dr. Smith that a new doctor in the Twin Cities would pick up where he left off, with surgery workup.

Hope is what I would cling to in the days and weeks ahead, hope that a team of medical experts could end the seizures that had ended my career. Perhaps being a reporter prepared me to handle this. A core trait of reporting is determination. We're used to sending multiple emails, making multiple calls, asking questions until we get the details we need. Sometimes we get put on hold or our calls go unanswered. We're naturally disappointed when stories fall through; when a yes turns to a no; or, worse, when a no from the start never changes, even with more effort. But in reporting, the effort was always worth it when the story came through. The medical and legal calls I was making now were no different. My post-reporting phase was being measured in paperwork: unemployment forms, job applications, and medical forms.

The beautiful greenery outside my window was the one thing that brought some calm as I alternated between sitting and standing, moving from one phone call to the next. Spacious grounds surrounded my apartment building, and every window overlooked dozens of bright green trees, with a pond right outside my patio window. In late July and August, the sunny skies and sounds of geese honking and flocking about drew my gaze when I would lose my focus on the daunting tasks in front of me.

Finally, ten days after sending my email to the Epilepsy Foundation, I received a phone call. A representative with the Epilepsy Legal Defense Fund told me a local employment attorney was willing to look at my case. Named to honor attorney Jeanne A. Carpenter, the fund aims to end epilepsy-related discrimination through public education and access to legal services.

The attorney offered to work pro bono to see if I had a potential case. I couldn't believe my luck. I requested my personnel files from the TV station right away. A Michigan law called the Bullard-Plawecki Employee Right to Know Act required my boss to share my personnel records.

Never in my life did I dread a piece of mail arriving as much as that document. A small envelope arrived in the mail a couple days later. I dropped it onto my kitchen table and stared at it for a few seconds. What was in there? It wasn't large enough to cover my nearly three years at the station, which I had requested. Tension quickly filled my body as I sat down, picked up the envelope, and slowly opened it. A few words made clear what I was about to read. In my hands were notes from my boss's investigation with my colleague about the seizure.

My mind rewound to what I told Ann that day in her office:

"I don't want to know, not if it gets worse."

When she had started explaining the details, I asked her to stop. Comprehending what she was saying at the time was impossible. Now the "worse" was right here in my hands. I wanted to shred the papers, but at this point, I needed to know more, to understand what this seizure had done to me.

Cautiously, I opened the first page, caught a quick glimpse of my name, and closed it again.

You'll be fine. Just read it.

After taking a deep breath, I turned the page and read a few sentences, and my chin and stomach immediately dropped to the floor.

I inhaled quickly and looked away, bewildered, then tried to catch my breath.

No, I can't read anymore, can't do this, can't do this, can't do this to myself.

But I needed to know how it ends.

Scrolling toward the bottom, I caught the words "psychotic episode" on the way down.

Psychotic episode? That's how my colleague described my seizure?!
I lost it.

"I'm not psychotic; it was a seizure!" I yelled at the words staring back at me.

I started to cry.

"That wasn't the real me!"

I stuffed the document haphazardly back into the envelope and pushed it across the table. There was no way I could read anymore.

"Why would she say that?"

My sense of self-worth plummeted, and I sank down in my chair, trying to push "psychotic episode" out of my mind. Never had I wanted to forget anything more.

Please forget that. You have forgotten so many wonderful memories, please, please erase this one, the worst one.

I needed something to distract me, so I glanced across the room. Boxes. They littered the space in front of my couch. My parents would be here in a few days, and I still had packing to do. There was no time to sit and dwell on a few sentences.

18

Coming Home and Reaching
New Heights

When moving day finally arrived, my head turned for one last check around my empty apartment, and my eyes shifted slowly from the kitchen to the living room. Never again would I walk by every spot where a seizure had struck, or recall the déjà vu when opening my closet, or gaze blankly at the pictures on the wall and the appliances in the kitchen. I was grateful to shut the door on that part of my life and turn over the key, locking inside almost three years of physical and emotional pain those blackouts had caused. On July 22, the door to my career was effectively slammed shut in my face. Now I hoped the Twin Cities would open a new door.

My parents hitched up the U-Haul trailer and we headed west. Highway 196 hugs the Lake Michigan shore, and we traveled around the lake and into Chicago. We drove past the city, up through Madison, Wisconsin, and a few hours later the setting sun glowed over the skyline ahead. Minnesota's capital city came into view. The drive brought me back to college, a time when cruising along the interstate was carefree. But now I was a passenger. One of the most frustrating parts of epilepsy was losing the freedom to sit in the driver's seat.

One exit we flew by that night would soon become a familiar and important one. A few blocks off of I-94 in Saint Paul stood the John Nasseff Neuroscience Specialty Clinic, home of the Minnesota Epilepsy Group. Connected to the clinic was United Hospital, and I would soon get to know both places very well.

We continued the drive and turned the corner into a southwest Minneapolis neighborhood about twenty minutes later. My college friend Christine was renting her coworker's house, and they were looking for another roommate. Living with an old college friend was exactly what I needed.

With my new life ahead of me, the possibility of brain surgery was at the top of my mind. Although I knew absolutely nothing about the surgery or its risks yet, I was already willing to do whatever was necessary to get my life back.

The meeting with my new doctor was still two months away, and with the risks and uncertainty ahead, I was getting restless. I had never had any real downtime in my life. My mind wandered, wondering if I could put life on pause to run away to another country for a few weeks. The idea had first crossed my mind in Michigan, when I needed mental breaks from the tasks at hand to avoid a breakdown. Now the timing was ideal. The best thing physically, emotionally, and mentally for me would be to take a trip. My curiosity led me to a group adventure in New Zealand with other young travelers.

The photos online sold me. Nothing else could get my mind off my brain, so I convinced myself that white-water rafting, snorkeling with dolphins, and bungee jumping would do it. The mental escape became real once I grasped how much I truly needed this—I didn't even think twice about bungee jumping.

Nor did I think twice about the possibility of having seizures half a world away or what kind of medical care would be there. The worst had already happened, I believed, so nothing could go wrong on a vacation. If anyone tried to convince me to stay home, I brushed them off. Looking back, in my desperation for a change of scenery, I was obviously in denial about the possibility of future seizures. Traveling within the United States wouldn't satisfy me. And for some reason, the idea of visiting an island in the South Pacific, eight thousand miles from home, didn't worry me in the slightest.

A spot was still open for the early October adventure. I could also visit someone on the way there. My sister had known me longer than anyone and knew how much I needed to get away. I called Sara to set a date, bought a one-way ticket to San Francisco, and then booked my trip to New Zealand. I sat back and smiled;

this was possibly the most spontaneous thing I'd ever done. Two months later, I packed my bags to the max and boarded a plane to California. Once the wheels pushed off the runway, I let out the breath I'd been holding tight in my chest for weeks. A few hours later, Sara greeted me at the airport with a huge hug and a smile. "I'm so lucky to have you," I said with gratitude.

She helped me roll my luggage over to the subway, and we headed to the house she shared with friends and made dinner.

"I want you to get your mind off what happened by changing your environment," she told me. "I want you to wake up at sunrise with me and walk up to the top of Twin Peaks to see the view. I want everything to feel normal and to feel secure."

It took leaving the Midwest for me to finally feel like things might actually turn out OK. This was my third trip to the city, but Twin Peaks was a first. Early one morning we bundled up and headed toward the two hills with 360-degree panoramic views of San Francisco, the bay, and the ocean. I smile now thinking of this moment because I can recall it completely. An orange glow slowly rose above us as we hiked up the half mile of terrain, where fog greeted us at the top. The low-lying haze cast a magical view over the city and the surrounding water. Suddenly, everything felt OK. Standing on a giant hill in California with my sister, two thousand miles from home, truly did make my problems seem far away.

That calm, scenic morning set the tone for the next few days. My work and health problems stayed in the background, helping me focus solely on Sara and San Francisco. As sisters, though, we were bound to disagree on something after spending time together. Toward the end of my visit, we got into an argument. I don't remember the details, but Sara said I was flustered and left her house to go for a run. It never occurred to her that running in an unfamiliar place was a risk for me.

Taking off in one direction and coming back via the same route would make it impossible to get lost. But my plan didn't work out. A seizure struck, and I lost awareness. Once my world came back in focus, my sense of direction had vanished.

Where am I?

That all too familiar question filled my thoughts once again. But this time, I didn't even remember that I was in San Francisco. My dad recalls this seizure, because for some reason I called him in Minnesota.

He could tell by my nervous tone that I was lost.

"You're in San Francisco visiting Sara," he said, concerned. "Go into the nearest shop to ask them where you are." Then he gave me Sara's address.

I had my sister's address in my phone somewhere, but with my consciousness impaired, my brain was still foggy, and I had no clue where to look for it. My dad walked me through the steps to find my way back.

An hour later, I walked up the steps to Sara's house.

"I feel terrible," she told me and gave me a hug.

Just a few minutes later, my brain turned on me.

"While we were talking in my bedroom, your eyes got wide and you started waving your arms in a wingspan," Sara recalled, "walking toward me and making inaudible noises. I realized I was witnessing a large seizure for the first time, not an aura like in the past. I didn't know what to do or if I should talk to you or touch your arm."

"It was scary to look into the eyes of my sister and see someone I didn't recognize," she explained. "When you snapped out of it, you were really confused. It was shortly before your college roommate and track teammate Joellen had arranged to come over to meet us for dinner. You wanted to calm down a bit more before seeing a friend you hadn't seen in a while, but you were clearly confused. You repeated questions and didn't remember details about your time together in college. Joellen looked to me for clues and to understand your confusion."

Not a single moment from Joellen's visit comes back to me. Another vacation moment lost, another reason to consider surgery.

In retrospect, that seizure should have made me think twice about New Zealand, but it didn't. Instead, I looked past the danger toward what I could do differently. That run reinforced the importance of replacing worries with sleep if I wanted to have fun in New Zealand. That's easier said than done, but I made the decision to enjoy the present instead of dwelling on seizures. Sara hugged me tight at the airport a few days later. I wasn't about to cloud my vision of gorgeous mountains and waterfalls with the uncertainty ahead of me. I can't recall if I told the flight crew or my trip guides of my epilepsy, but I hope I was responsible enough to do so.

When my plane landed, twenty-five fellow adventure seekers from across the world greeted me with excited hellos. We were all in our late twenties or early thirties and hopped on a tour bus to spend the next two weeks climbing, jumping, diving, and pushing ourselves to the limit. I took as many photos as possible, knowing the likelihood of remembering the vacation was slim. I had never approached a vacation with that mindset, but there was nothing I could deny anymore.

We hiked up and through the challenging, snow-packed terrain of Mount Tongariro in Tongariro National Park. Then we grabbed our ice picks and sledded with cautious excitement to the bottom. The snow would often be replaced by warm sun and sand in a single day. The North Face logos adorned nearly every layer I wore.

We rafted down a steep drop and bounced into the Tongariro River. We jumped into the pristine blue Bay of Islands to snorkel alongside coral fish, seahorses, and turtles. Mud slathered my skin in a bath at Hell's Gate, an active geothermal reserve. And on the last day of the trip, I found the guts to check something off my bucket list.

Our bus traveled sixty miles south to Taupo. Right outside the small city, we pulled up to the Waikato River, New Zealand's longest, bordered by massive rock formations and green trees on both sides. I stepped out and looked up to see a huge wooden platform overlooking the beautiful blue winding river, one of the images that had inspired me to sign up for the trip. Two people with white helmets walked tentatively to the platform in their bungee harnesses. My heart rate spiked immediately as they approached the edge of the platform, and right when the tandem prepared to jump, I looked away. Watching someone jump over an unforgiving river was too scary.

But a few seconds later, the sound of terrified screams briefly filled the air, and we walked closer to see the jumpers dangling from the cord with big smiles. Their adrenaline rush convinced me to climb the rocks to the platform with my group, but when I took one look down at the water my heart rate spiked again. The photos online made it look like the most exciting thing in the world. But signing up online and signing my life away on the liability papers were two different things. Two of my new friends planned a tandem jump, and my body tensed as they took deep breaths, waved goodbye with nervous smiles, and then turned and leaped from the platform. Now it was my turn. The instructor strapped me into the harness and guided me to the edge. I shifted hesitantly side to side as he carefully attached the long cord to the harness.

"All set!" he smiled encouragingly.

I looked at him, glanced down, and stepped back from the jump spot. There was no way in hell I was jumping the height of a twelve-story building.

But peer pressure is strong on trips like this.

Logic also reminded me that I had already paid and would look like a fool by backing out. So I stepped out of my comfort zone and back onto the platform, shifting my weight and peeking down below again. The air was silent. After ten seconds or so, the instructor offered to push me off. That was my only other option now—jump or be pushed.

"No, no, no. I'll jump!"

And before I could change my mind again, I leaped off the platform, shrieking as the harness rotated me headfirst, and I went spiraling straight down toward the river. My voice was muffled by the wind, and I instinctively tucked my chin into my neck to hide the view of the water as it drew closer and closer. The descent was over in seconds. I opened my eyes cautiously, thankful that I was indeed still alive, upside down, slowly drifting side to side and staring straight into clear blue water. I started laughing. All the anxiety that went into this jump, only for it to end so quickly. Bungee jumping was not the exhilarating moment I had imagined, but it was definitely an adrenaline rush. Then it hit me.

Two weeks of adventure a world away, capped off by bungee jumping, was the best self-help therapy available. Not one seizure had struck. The mix of fun, terror, excitement, and conversations with interesting travelers on the island erased the stress and insomnia that my job and epilepsy caused at the time. The photos in my album show it clearly. Genuine smiles fill each one, without a trace of worry across my face.

I had the time of my life in New Zealand with some awesome people—that I remember with clarity—but within a few months, highlights from the trip started to disappear. What island was I on? Where did we snorkel and white-water raft? What were the names of my fellow travelers? In time, everything disappeared, except for bungee jumping.

That moment remains the only memory from the trip that I can recall, detail by detail. Every detail I describe in the other photos is what I know I did, but I don't remember the actual experience. The bus rides, the conversations, where we slept each night and ate each day—these are also a blank slate.

The picture of me sledding down the steep, snow-packed mountain looks like a freeze frame of a scene in an adventure movie. The viewer has a hint of what is going to happen but doesn't know the outcome. As I look through my photos, every moment on the trip except for bungee jumping is a freeze frame. Why is it that certain moments from losing my job are ingrained in my mind, while memories of the best adventures of my life vanished within a few months?

19

Stigma, Up Close and Personal

Sun streamed in through the high windows, casting shadows over treadmills and stationary bikes. Though it was early spring, winter still held its grip on the weather, and black ice covered some of the roads. A warm, cozy gym would have to do for now. One afternoon, I jumped on a bike facing a wall with a window above. After about ten minutes, my view narrowed, and tunnel vision set in. My stomach sank.

Oh no, no, no. Please don't be an aura. Please don't.

The strange feeling persisted, and I should have listened to the warning and left the gym immediately. But the seizure moved quickly and overtook me.

The next thing I remember is regaining awareness, somewhat dizzy, exhausted, but still pedaling away. I pulled my feet to a stop and sat there for a moment, well aware of a woman's eyes on me. She was exercising five feet away. I stood up and caught her stare, one of great concern. She didn't look much older than me.

"You were biking and just started screaming," she told me.

Embarrassed, I nodded.

"Yes, that was a seizure. I'm sorry it scared you."

The surprise and concern didn't leave her face as I quickly said goodbye and headed for the door, my head down. But a bald, middle-aged man stopped me before I could leave.

"You were on that bike screaming. You were just screaming," he said in a hostile tone.

"Yes, that was a seizure," I repeated. "I'm sorry it scared you."

He asked if I was religious, a Christian, and then told me: "You must have a multiple personality disorder."

My mouth dropped. How could I even respond to such ignorance?

I've always been someone to stick up for myself. Even as a young child, my mom said I made a boy cry when he tried to bully me at our neighborhood pool. Reporters take a lot of crap in the field and from viewers, so we tend to develop a thick skin. But that comment was unlike anything I'd ever heard; it almost left me speechless.

"No," I responded firmly. "It was a seizure."

I didn't expect him to know that certain parts of speech and movement are controlled by the frontal lobe and that if neurons are misfiring there, a person may start yelling and waving their arms in circles. But I did expect a grown adult to be respectful and not jump to conclusions. His cruel comment just furthered the stigma of mental illness and epilepsy.

The man shook his head, with a doubtful "yeah, right" expression, and didn't apologize. I held his stare for a second, then walked out the door in disbelief.

"You must have a multiple personality disorder."

Wow.

I had come face-to-face with stigma, and it stung. It stung hard enough to leave me at a loss for words, when usually I'd stand up for myself.

Nearly three million people in the United States live with epilepsy, and many have encountered ignorance like this. Who else had this man insulted? Until that day, I hadn't realized how lucky I'd been. Most people who witnessed one of my seizures for the first time came to my side, soothed me, and reoriented me no matter how many times I asked the day or time. They included my coworkers and strangers at makeup counters and in airports.

At that moment I decided I wouldn't waste any more time feeling self-conscious about having epilepsy. There was no reason to let an asshole at the gym make me feel inferior. Yes, seizures can be scary to witness, but once people understand how they form, they can help increase awareness and offer empathy. I knew then that the social stigma surrounding epilepsy wasn't something that could be easily solved.

On October 20, 2014, it was time to meet my new epileptologist, Dr. Patricia Penovich at the Minnesota Epilepsy Group. The high ceilings and windows of the John Nasseff Neuroscience Specialty Clinic brought an immediate calm, making me forget for a second that I was there to see a doctor. My mom and I made our way to the second floor, where a receptionist greeted us, and a nurse soon arrived to take us into an exam room. Dr. Penovich walked in a short while later with a bright smile and introduced herself. She had a sense of calm authority and years of experience, and I warmed to her right away. Brain surgery came into the discussion early, and once she knew I was interested, she got the ball rolling.

My epilepsy was very likely drug-resistant by then, also called intractable. Two drugs had failed to control the seizures, which is the first criteria for surgery consideration. The next step was finding out where the seizures were firing from, to determine what kind of surgery would be possible.

There are three broad types of epilepsy surgery—resective, disconnective, and neuromodulatory—and within each category there are many different procedures. Resective surgery is the removal of a small portion of the brain, and it is only possible when seizures are firing from one identifiable spot. In disconnective surgery, nerve fibers are severed to interrupt the spread of seizures from one hemisphere to the other. In neuromodulatory surgery, a medical device is implanted that uses electrical impulses to shorten the length, number, and severity of seizures.

Deep brain stimulation, responsive neurostimulation, and vagal nerve stimulation are devices used in people with epilepsy.

The outcome for epilepsy surgery is good for some types of surgery, but not as great for others. Resections are the most invasive procedures, but they have the best long-term outcome. The most common epilepsy resective surgery in adults with a high success rate is a cortico-amygdalohippocampectomy. It treats seizures forming in one of the temporal lobes.

Prior EEGs had confirmed I had focal epilepsy in my right hemisphere, which made me a potential candidate for a resection. That was the good news. We just didn't know yet whether the seizures were firing from the frontal or temporal lobe. To get started,

Dr. Penovich scheduled another round of video EEG testing in the hospital. That surprised me.

"Can't you use the video EEG from Dr. Smith in Michigan?"

"No," she smiled. She wanted her own.

OK. Whatever it took to find answers, I agreed to.

Surgery candidacy for epilepsy was much more complex than I anticipated or understood. Several tests were required to determine if I would be eligible. Doctors first needed a baseline to see how my brain was currently operating, and they needed evidence that my brain was in fact dysfunctioning and where. The "where" part was very important. Surgeons wouldn't risk disrupting areas of the brain that control crucial functions like language and speech, so the results of my tests would determine whether I got a green light or a red light for the next step—surgery to map my brain.

Over the next four months, I would meet with two neuropsychologists, a psychologist, a cardiologist, another epileptologist, and a physical therapist. Everyone played important roles, and each person brought me a step closer to a cure. I was grateful that Dr. Penovich had put such a comprehensive plan in place, and for the first time since my 2013 video EEG testing in Michigan, I felt optimistic.

The same day that Dr. Penovich was writing up plans for my surgery workup, the head of labor relations at my former TV station was drafting a letter with the rest of my personnel file. I was at my friend's house searching for jobs, and seeing his name in my email inbox made me jump.

I took a deep breath and clicked on the attachment, my finger shaking so much it took three attempts to press hard enough for the PDF document to open. The page count took me by surprise. Seventy-three pages. It was my entire work file, not just the notes about my termination and epilepsy. My fingers started to scroll. The first email regarding epilepsy started four pages in with a letter from Dr. Smith notifying my boss, Ann, that I couldn't drive.

The next email came as a surprise, but maybe it shouldn't have. A coworker had emailed Ann to voice concerns that I was forgetting things and not taking her advice to help me remember them. Next up was the seizure action plan Ann put together. Every single email between us was attached.

"Stacia, I heard you had another seizure . . ."

We put a lot of effort into forming that plan, and she was supportive, which made reading it at that moment too hard. My eyes stayed glued to the screen as I scrolled down, hoping with each passing page that I wouldn't run into something else critical of my performance. But then appeared another producer's critique of my inability to drive.

Sitting there, my mind wandered for a bit.

If I was healthy and didn't have epilepsy, would I ever write to my boss a critical message about someone who did have epilepsy? Of course not. People with epilepsy can't stop their neurons from misfiring at will.

Then came the internal emails and dictated discussions about that awful day. I skimmed them over, looking for details I either didn't remember or didn't know about. Soon I landed on the page when Ann started reciting the allegations. My throat went dry. I quickly clicked out of the document and closed my email. Emotionally, I wasn't ready to go back there, but now I truly knew how much epilepsy had impacted my career.

20

Black and White

Don't open it. Don't.

My curiosity convinced me I'd be fine. Months had passed, after all. I was visiting my parents in Thief River Falls, and for reasons unknown today, I thought it would be a good idea to look back at the summer day in 2014 when my career ended.

With an anxious flutter in my chest, I climbed the stairs to my bedroom and approached my closet where I was keeping most of my belongings until I found a permanent place to live. Inside a locked box on the ground was my personnel file, my termination letter, and a document that detailed the July 22 seizures. My fingers shook as I fumbled with the key, opened the box, and pulled out the papers. Their weight and texture immediately clicked in my brain.

You read through some of this once, and nothing has changed. What are you looking for this time?

Peace. Peace of mind. No matter how difficult it will be to read, I need to confront this so I don't ever think of it again.

First, the termination letter. Ann had read it aloud to me, but it had all blurred together. My pulse had already quickened when I plopped down on the carpet in the middle of my room.

There it was in black and white: "your last day . . . your conduct . . . so were [sic] are terminating you effective immediately." The grammatical error felt like an ironic ending to my journalism career as I knew it.

The words stung more on paper. What had blurred together when she spoke was now clear as day in print. The words "your conduct" glared back at me, a reminder of a year earlier, when the same words played like a broken record in my mind.

Hot tears started flowing.

"Why does it say 'your'!" I cried out at that piece of paper. "Epilepsy did that, not me!"

If she had replaced "your" with "epilepsy" and written "the reason for this action is what epilepsy caused your body to do," I might have handled it a little better. Maybe. My cotton shirt proved to be the perfect clothing for today, as I wiped my tears on one of the sleeves, then peered down at the other document on the floor. It stared back at me, warning, "Don't open me. Don't."

But I had to at that point. The small section I had read in my Michigan apartment was not the entire story, and the stress had erased what I did read from my memory. My hands started to tremble as soon as I picked up the next document, and my fingers slowly turned to the first page. At the top, my name, and underneath, the words my brain had intentionally forgotten in order to save me from this feeling again. I scanned the letter, turning away as the memory resurfaced. Forcing myself to look back at what I skipped, I read another sentence in disbelief. Then the words "psychotic episode" reappeared and my stomach sank.

My shaky hands dropped the paper, and I spotted the termination letter. The anger, hurt, and humiliation building in my chest soon overflowed, and I started ripping the papers up, all of them, into tiny pieces as quickly as possible. But random words still stared back at me from the pile at my feet, so I jumped up to grab a scissors from my desk and sliced through each word, each and every letter on paper now so small it fell like snow falling from my trembling fingers. Once I could no longer see the hurtful words, I dropped the scissors and sat back on my heels, surrounded by shredded paper so fine that restructuring a sentence would have been impossible. But all my efforts couldn't erase the vision of the words "psychotic episode" and "your conduct" next to my name.

"You, you, you, Stacia, are a horrible, shameful person" is what those words said to me.

I wanted them to slide from my thoughts and drown. I wanted them gone forever, never to reappear. But the idea of those words sitting in my parents' garbage overwhelmed me.

With the bag of shredded paper in hand, I flew downstairs to the kitchen, opened the first drawer that might contain matches, and dug around in it. Nothing. Onto the next drawer, nothing. Onto the next drawer, and there they were. The fireplace had zero wood, and just thinking about a fire inside on this warm spring day made me sweat. The view outside the kitchen window showed me my options. My eyes darted back and forth and landed on our concrete driveway behind the house on the alley. A tall fence provided cover from the next-door neighbor.

Good enough. Tears fell as I flew open the back door to the garage. I jumped back in surprise to see the large garage door open and my mom packing up boxes. I sailed by her without a word and headed to the side of the house with a cement strip and the tall fence. No one could see me here.

I clutched the tiny box of matches in one shaking hand, the shredded paper in the other. Never in my life had burning anything come to mind, but never in my life had anything upset me this much. I was nearly hyperventilating as I bent down to press the shredded paper into a mound on the cement, thankful the winds were calm.

It was impossible to tell *b* from *d*, and *t* from *f*, because they were sliced and diced to obliteration. No matter. Placing one foot over the paper mound to keep it in place, I propped myself up, took out a match, and clumsily struck at the stripe on the box.

Please light, please light, please light.

Whoosh.

A flame came to life.

My heavy breathing nearly blew the match out, so I swiveled my head left, took a deep breath, and turned back to the flame. A short circuit in my brain had sparked the storm that caused the actions described on this paper. Now a spark would destroy those words. I had to see the reason I was terminated on fire. My heart raced as I bent down to set the tiny letters ablaze, then stood up quickly to see black and white dissolve into ash.

"That's not me, that's not me!!"

My voice cried as I stomped my feet over the fire.

The flames erased the words, but not the shame. I needed

someone to explain why epilepsy was guilty, not me. How could a brain go from holding an ordinary conversation to having a total collapse of judgment in a matter of seconds?

The smell of smoke didn't take long to travel. My mom caught a whiff and ran out of the garage in panic.

"Stacia! What are you doing? You can't burn something so close to the house!"

"I don't care!" I cried. "I cannot see those words again! I didn't do this! Why would I do this? This isn't me!"

My sobbing escalated. She tried to soothe me, but she had never seen me so upset. I'd never seen myself so upset. Completely inconsolable, I quickly sailed back into the house while my mom made sure the flames were completely out. Then she came in to check on me, but she knew from previous experience that it was best to leave me alone and let me work through things on my own. She stopped in her tracks, unsure of what to do.

My body paced back and forth in the kitchen, trying to distract my brain from those words. How does someone decide to correlate a seizure with a psychotic episode? I realized the only person who could possibly comfort me at that point was in Michigan. The hours of Googling medical papers hadn't given me concrete answers. The internet was no substitute for a human being. My hands, still shaking, scrolled through names on my phone. There he was: Dr. Smith. In my experience, doctors rarely take patient calls, but I was desperate.

Wait, calm down first. You sound like a train wreck.

After a few long deep breaths, my finger hit the call button, then followed a few prompts. His nurse answered. My emotions started to bubble up again, and the hyperventilating returned.

"Can I talk to Dr. Smith?"

I don't remember what I said next, but my tone must have gotten the message across. After a short hold, he came on the phone. His voice was the warm, friendly tone I knew from the clinic. Everything inside me started spilling out.

"Why, why, why would I do that??" I cried. "How could I possibly have interacted with another person during a seizure?? I've never done that before!"

He gently explained that it wasn't my fault. His tone was relaxed and matter-of-fact.

"You didn't do that because 'Oh, I'm going to have a seizure and this is what I want to do.' No," he said. "Remember, you don't have the conscious level that you're making decisions on your behavior."

That would also be true if the behavior had happened during the postictal state and not during the seizure.

Epilepsy is black-and-white when it comes to motive. I stopped pacing and sat down at the kitchen island. My breathing finally started to slow down as he explained everything, and my humiliation started to wane.

I knew for certain that I didn't know what happened, but in that moment, I needed to hear Dr. Smith's reassurance again. Relieved and grateful, I hung up the phone. This was the second time Dr. Smith had taken my call, and it showed his humanity as a doctor. The first call from my boss's office in Michigan and now this one from my parents' house were two of the most important phone calls of my life. I'd never experienced something I couldn't work out on my own until now.

Each time was a crisis call for help, and hearing his helpful voice on the other end meant the world to me. What would have happened if he hadn't taken the call that day? Epilepsy had taken control of my life in many ways, but I had always been able to control my emotions to some extent. When Ann relayed some of the accusations to me in her office, I broke down and asked her to speak to Dr. Smith, but I was still able to pull myself together, walk home, sort out my emotions, and calm down.

Today was different. There was something different about seeing those horrible words in print versus hearing them out loud. For me, spoken words are much easier to forget, even more so in a state of shock when everything blends together in a flash.

But print is permanent and gives you the option to see the words over and over again and come back to them a year later. Some parts of the past are not meant to be revisited. Ironically in that moment, I needed to destroy any chance of remembering.

If that fits the description of a mental breakdown, there it is. Life had kept me so busy—the attorney, the move to Minnesota, my new doctor, the New Zealand trip, the surgery workup—that hurt had to be pushed aside. A few medical professionals have asked if I became depressed after I was terminated or after I saw the termination file. Depression and anxiety are common in temporal lobe epilepsy, and an unsuccessful surgery could make symptoms worse. For this reason, I was scheduled to see a psychologist to make a thorough evaluation of my mental health.

After I was fired, I couldn't get past feeling like a bad person. The humiliation was real. But depressed? No, I didn't feel depressed. Talking with Dr. Smith had erased all the doubt and anguish that seeing those words in print had provoked. Nobody else could take away my doubt at that time. With his reassurance, I could finally move on.

21

A Battery of Tests

Some people hate hospitals. I've never been one of those people. To me, hospitals represent hope, and as I walked toward the John Nasseff Neuroscience Specialty Clinic in Saint Paul for my first test, my chest was full of it.

This mid-November morning in 2014 would be day one of many visits. First up on the surgery workup was an intense test of brain power. No joke. A complex neuropsychology assessment used to evaluate brain function would test my smarts: my working memory, spatial awareness, judgment, dexterity, abstract reasoning, problem-solving, hand strength, and more. One crucial step was to determine which part of my brain housed my verbal and visual memories. No two brains are the same.

I was greeted with nearly every brain game I could think of that morning. The games would test every nook and cranny where memory was stored. Memory isn't stored in just one region of the brain; it involves many areas and pathways. During the tests, I drew designs from memory (Wechsler Memory Scale test); identified line drawings of things like shoes, then said the word out loud (Boston Naming Test); traced through mazes (Porteus Maze); named colors (Delis-Kaplan Executive Function System test); matched flashcards by color, shape, or number (Wisconsin Card Sorting Test); and more.

Some verbal tests entailed retrieving memories of things I should have known, like words that start with t. Easy. Tom came to mind first, then Tennessee. But then I was told I couldn't say names or states. Shoot. "Tyrannosaurus rex," I blurted out, then laughed. The randomness of my answer surprised me. The neuropsychologist asked me to remember a mix of random words, repeat them thirty seconds later, and then recall them again a few minutes after that. I mentally grouped the words, hoping that correlating them to something would help me recall them, and the result was pretty good. Though I don't recall the specific questions on that day, the exams often included a fruit, the name of a state, and a color.

Then came the drawings. To test my visual memory, the examiner showed me a handful of different designs, one at a time, for a short period, then took them away and asked me to draw each from memory. I focused hard to snap a mental picture of the entire shape, then to catch a quick detail or two. As the examiner pulled the picture away, though, most of my memory went along with it. I could usually hang onto one detail to draw and sometimes sketch a decent outline, but everything between the lines was a blur and only got blurrier as the test progressed. Sometimes I'd catch only a frame of the new photo before me but remember something from a previous one and then create a hybrid drawing.

Another test presented a grid with marked locations and simple designs placed in each spot. Once it was taken away, I had to place the designs on the grid. The grid game quickly became overwhelming, and I felt as though my eyes were playing tricks on me.

How can I forget something so quickly?

I asked myself this over and over.

Instead of getting frustrated, I tried to observe what I simply couldn't do well, joking that a kindergartener could probably do a better job. It would have been very interesting to compare my memory at that time with someone my age who didn't have epilepsy and also compare it to my own memory from five years earlier. Since I'm not an artist, maybe my sketching was always haphazard, I reasoned, reassuring myself.

More activities filled the day, and brain drain started to set in. It was a sprint rather than a marathon version of cramming for a test in college, except the material was everything I had learned in elementary school—shapes, colors, drawing, and simple vocabulary. Instead of staying up all night to force a semester's worth of content into my memory bank for one big test, I crammed in dozens of mini exams, one after another, to recall thirty seconds later and then again a few hours later. They weren't complex physics equations, but the sheer scope of material was daunting.

The testing results revealed clear deficits in my visual memory, which is the ability to recall what you've seen recently and long-term: faces, buildings, or pictures in a magazine. The neuropsychologist said that, overall, my results were generally consistent with right temporal abnormality, meaning my right temporal lobe wasn't functioning normally.

How much worse could this inevitably get if seizures continued? Was it hard to predict?

She noted that I had slow reaction time and slow psychomotor speed, which is the time it takes someone to process new information, comprehend it, and physically respond.

Dr. Penovich suspected one of my medications, Zonisamide, could be causing this, so she took me off it and started me on a new ASM, Vimpat. I retook part of the test a month later, and my reaction time improved. I figured that Zonisamide had probably impacted my reporting abilities.

Vimpat was the ASM that Dr. Kiley had initially wanted me to try in Oregon, but it was too expensive at the time. I hoped Vimpat would be the answer, but it didn't take long for a seizure to strike. My faith in medication all but disappeared at that point; three medications had failed.

The battery of tests that day showed clear deficits, but they didn't capture the entire picture of my brain function. My creative side—shooting and editing video—was stronger than ever; a compilation of my best video journalism work from 2014 was nominated for a Michigan Emmy Award. In a year of bad news, this felt pretty good.

More psychological and memory testing would come, but next up was test number two, a magnetoencephalography (MEG). Like the EEG, an MEG measures brain activity, but this test gives a near instantaneous high-resolution recording of the electrical currents inside neurons. It detects spikes in brain waves more precisely than the EEG. The test took only two hours, and it confirmed that my left hemisphere was dominant for speech and language, which is true for most people. The distinction between the two is important. Language is stored in the dominant temporal lobe and is the ability to understand the meaning of words to form sentences, while speech is stored in the dominant frontal lobe and is the ability to form sounds, speak fluently, and articulate ideas. To understand language and be able to speak, the dominant frontal and temporal lobes need to interact.

So far so good. Surgery would be a no-go if it would impact my language, speech, and other critical functions. My heart was now standing in the way of what is typically the quickest test for surgery workup. Remember, my heart's electrical system was also dysfunctional, and a pacemaker was keeping my heartbeat at a steady rhythm. An echocardiogram had confirmed that my heart was working properly, and a physical therapist's observation of me biking for fifteen minutes didn't show anything concerning.

So what was the problem? The pacemaker itself.

The small, oval-shaped titanium device was preventing Dr. Penovich from finding out if there was damaged tissue in my brain that could be causing the seizures. An MRI shows clear images of brain tissue, and a lesion would show up as a bright spot. The issue was that pacemakers aren't usually allowed near MRI machines because the strong magnetic field can trigger changes in the settings of the heart device. The only solution was to swap it out with an MRI-compatible pacemaker.

So, on a frigid mid-December day, I checked into the Nasseff Heart Center at United Hospital. The building was familiar to me by now because my epilepsy clinic was right next door. Enough had happened with my brain in the last five months that my heart felt like an afterthought. A new pacemaker seemed like the easiest item to check off the list. I changed into a hospital gown and traded in my snow boots for cozy hospital slippers.

The surgeon removed the little box—called the pulse generator—and replaced it with the MRI-compatible one. He also inserted two new wires into one of my heart's chambers and connected them to the pulse generator. Thankfully, no blood clots formed this time. The actual MRI would be a few weeks later. Up next was another round of video EEG monitoring.

During all the surgery workup, there was one thing I didn't have trouble remembering. My attorney was reviewing my case, and I was trying to be patient. Then, two days before my video EEG monitoring, he contacted me.

He could not find any decisions from cases involving epilepsy but did come across a case in another jurisdiction with an analogous scenario involving an employee with a disability. In that case, the court ruled that an employer does not have to tolerate or allow the conduct as part of its duty to accommodate.

Would a court in Michigan rule that my situation was comparable to the situation in that case?

My mind raced to come up with some kind of counterargument. What about this? Or that?

But I had a bad feeling that the answer would be yes.

Defeated, I thanked him for working so hard to help, hung up the phone, and sat down at the counter, trying to absorb everything. What else could I do? I hung my head in disappointment.

But now came the question, Should I get a second opinion from another employment attorney?

It was eating me up inside. Big questions ordinarily prompt me to get out a notepad and create a pros and cons list. My brain was busting out cons before the pen even hit the paper, cons I hadn't fully considered with my attorney because my focal point was discrimination. Ink was filling the page, but it couldn't keep up with my brain, spitting out con after con.

Could I handle walking back into the same courthouse where I had suffered a seizure to listen to my former colleague describe what had happened that day, with no way of defending myself since I had lost all awareness?

Could I handle facing an attorney who knew nothing about me but nonetheless would try to destroy my character?

My head was in my hands, my palms pushing against my eyes to try and erase the image of me sitting in court.

Would Dr. Smith have to testify, and what would he say? Would the judge side with a prominent Michigan epileptologist or the TV station? My only argument—that I would never, ever do something like that, that I couldn't even comprehend it—would probably fall on deaf ears. That was my gut feeling.

All the seizures, injuries, lost memories, work mistakes, and embarrassing moments now felt like just a few bumps in a long winding road from Oregon to Michigan, all leading to this—a head-on collision.

Could I physically or emotionally handle all this, knowing that my epilepsy was now bad enough to warrant more serious treatment? *No, you can't. You know you can't.*

My inner voice was blunt and definitive, with no option to think it over.

This may sound like I simply gave up and didn't seek justice. But here's the thing—I'm a realist, and I don't base my decisions purely on emotion. I would have had to go up against a huge media company with an army of lawyers, and I had no clear understanding of what truly happened that day. It's hard to stick up for yourself when you don't know the true story. I weighed my emotional brain versus my logical brain. On the one hand, I could fight for myself and others, but on the other, lawyers cost money, and I didn't have a job. Flights to Grand Rapids were expensive, and renting a car wasn't possible.

Your chances of winning are slim. This will be stressful, you'll lose sleep over it, and you'll have seizures. There's no denying that. You'll only delay treating your epilepsy. Focus on fixing your brain.

Overall, the cons beat out the pros. So I made the decision right then to move on. My athlete's mentality had matured. I wasn't giving up on myself and backing down from a fight; I was taking in the reality and caring for myself. For the first time in my six-year battle with epilepsy, I was truly putting my health before my pride.

The following night, I stayed up as long as possible so I could be sleep deprived for the new round of testing. I entered United Hospital the next morning bleary-eyed, groggy, and anxious to find out if my doctors here would catch the same "bizarre, unique, and unusual" seizures that Dr. Smith had found just a year earlier.

Once I settled into my room, an EEG technician arrived with the electrodes and glued them to my scalp. I knew the drill. My sleep and medications were reduced, and now came the waiting game for my brain to get crabby. The best chance of capturing a seizure would once again be through exercise, so a nurse walked me to an adjacent room with a stationary bike. Sure enough, soon after I started pedaling, neurons started misfiring.

My mom could hear me having the seizure from down the hall and rushed into the room.

"They were awful," she later told me. "When you were on the bicycle, I experienced what this seizure looks like for the first time. It was SCARY. Personally, I found all of these seizures scary—like, how could the person I know and love produce behavior that frightened me to my core?"

She didn't tell me this at the time, of course. The worry lines on her face when I reentered reality in the hospital room were telling enough.

But the end results left doctors with some of the same questions raised in Michigan. Seizure activity was showing up in the same places as the Michigan study, but a focal point still couldn't be found, and, once again, muscle artifact—signals recorded by EEG but not generated by the brain—was a big reason for this.

Were these large, violent seizures starting in the frontal lobe and spreading? Or could they have been starting elsewhere and then spreading to the frontal lobe? I wondered if my main auras—déjà vu and jamais vu—gave my doctors any clues.

The MRI was the last test needed and had the potential to give us some answers. Soon, I was back at United Hospital, this time sliding into an MRI machine. Several structural abnormalities associated with epilepsy can show up on the scan, and hippocampal sclerosis is one of the most common. An injured hippocampus would likely appear atrophied and brighter. This would signal scarring in the hippocampus, and that area of damage is called a lesion. The presence of a lesion would make me a great candidate for surgery because surgeons would know exactly where to resect tissue.

The MRI scan of my brain came back.

The good news was there was no lesion. I had epilepsy with no known focus yet.

But that was also the bad news. Without a lesion, it would be difficult to know whether the hippocampus was truly the generator. My frontal lobe seemed to be the area creating all the havoc, based on testing, so perhaps that was the area to remove.

My doctors, my neuropsychologists, and two neurosurgeons held a small conference to discuss my video EEG, MEG, MRI, and neuropsychology results. They would determine if I would be a good candidate for brain surgery.

On February 12, 2015, Dr. Penovich invited me to the clinic to share their decision.

22

"You Are a Candidate"

On a blustery, cold February afternoon, my mom and I walked into the Minnesota Epilepsy Group clinic, anxious to find out if a resection was a yes or a no. But my mind was also focused on finding a full-time job. Being unemployed for the last seven months had me on edge. Reporting was all I knew, and losing my job didn't exactly set me up for future success, so I had been looking into other journalism opportunities. One hour before the appointment, I emailed my college journalism instructor, Ken Stone, about a job posting. Then I headed out the door.

A nurse ushered us into a patient room, and we nervously waited to hear the medical team's decision. Dr. Penovich soon walked in with her warm smile and sat down on the stool. I was seated in a chair next to her desk, with my mom off to the side. Our conversation was a blur, except for the part my ears had been carefully listening for:

"You are a candidate for surgery," Dr. Penovich said happily.

I drew in a huge breath as my face broke into a smile. The tension I had carried for the last seven months dissolved as I exhaled audibly. "Yay! Yes!" I laughed.

"You didn't even think it over," my mom later said.

I didn't think anyone did.

This was a chance for seizure freedom.

Being a candidate meant I had cleared a few important hurdles—all the tests indicated my seizures weren't interfering with crucial brain functions, including verbal memory. The EEG results showed that most seizure activity was spreading across my right frontal lobe, which made it a good area to potentially resect. But the problem with EEG recordings is that they only record from the scalp. The only way to truly pinpoint the seizures would be to open a piece of my skull, by way of a craniotomy, and place intracranial electrodes (iEEG) directly onto the surface of my brain to record seizures.

Surgeons wouldn't go through all this work just to find the seizure onset, though.

They needed to identify the entire epileptogenic zone (EZ). This is the area necessary for generating seizures. Both the seizure onset zone and the EZ had to be resected in order to have a good shot at long-term seizure freedom. iEEG would map precisely where the seizures were firing from and identify the EZ. Another brain mapping tool would identify exactly where my critical functions were stored—called "functional cortical stimulation"—something the neuropsychology test couldn't do. My doctors could then compare the two maps to see if the EZ overlapped with any important functions; if it did, I would likely suffer deficits if that tissue was removed. If my ability to walk, talk, write, hear, understand language, and more were in the path of electrical storms, the second surgery—a resection—wouldn't happen.

For now, I could only concentrate on Dr. Penovich's words.

"You are a candidate."

If she mentioned all the risks, like infection, brain damage, and memory loss, that day, I wasn't listening closely. If she had said the operating room was open that night, I would have happily skipped to it.

The thought of drilling into my head to remove the tiny part of my brain that had destroyed my career finally lifted the weight from my shoulders. Who would have thought that the startling reality of brain surgery could bring such comfort?

Instinctively I knew there was no guarantee that surgery would end my seizures. There are no guarantees with anything in life. Details and risks are things I usually pay attention to, but the only fact that mattered now was that I was officially a candidate for brain surgery. Yes, it was a gamble, but I knew my doctors wouldn't approve the first surgery if they had any serious doubts that I would qualify for the second one.

At this point I just assumed everyone who qualified for surgery had the same reaction that I did:

"I qualified! Amazing! Yes!"

But various doctors and patients I would later meet told me no, just a small fraction of eligible candidates do, in fact, say yes. I was floored to hear people usually said no to surgery. Some people struggle with uncontrollable seizures for years, and they depend heavily on their caregivers. When patients are given the option of surgery and a chance to gain independence for the first time, doctors tell me, the reality of losing the stability of a caregiver is scary enough for some to decline surgery. Some people fear the idea of removing brain tissue, and others want a trade-off—they'll only do surgery if it comes with the guarantee that they can stop their seizure medication.

In surveys noted in a research journal comparing people who said yes versus no to surgery, results showed several reasons why patients declined surgery. They were more anxious about surgery, were less bothered by their epilepsy (despite comparable severity), were less likely to listen to their doctors (and others), and had more comorbid psychiatric disease. Some patients also had a general mistrust of brain surgery, negative medical provider opinions of surgery, lack of correct information about the success rates and risks, and poor patient-physician relationships. On the other hand, patients who chose surgery tended to be more embarrassed by their seizures, more interested in being seizure free, and less anxious about specific aspects of surgery.

Seizure freedom rates vary by procedure, and MRI results and seizure history can affect the outcome. Surgery outcome is worse in patients who suffer a high number of seizures, especially generalized tonic-clonic seizures. Positive outcomes are highest for patients with hippocampal lesions on their MRI who undergo a cortico-amygdalohippocampectomy. Approximately two-thirds of patients remain seizure free twenty years after surgery. But a surgery deemed successful doesn't necessarily mean complete seizure freedom. In people who are losing awareness and sometimes experiencing secondary generalized seizures, doctors consider surgery a success if the big seizures end and just small focal aware seizures continue. This is true for 74 percent of patients twenty years after surgery.

People without hippocampal lesions, like me, who have a cortico-amygdalohippocampectomy have a 76 percent chance of experiencing complete seizure freedom and an 81 percent chance of experiencing only focal aware seizures in the first year. However, at seven years and beyond, complete seizure freedom falls to 47 percent, while a reduction in seizures falls to 69 percent.

My tests results were leading doctors to a possible resection in my frontal lobe, where about 24 percent of patients become completely seizure free and 57 percent continue to have focal aware seizures at the seven-year mark.

So, there it was: My chance for seizure freedom long-term after undergoing a risky surgery was less than 50 percent. Less than half.

Would my glass be half empty or half full?

Wayne Gretzky said, "You miss 100 percent of the shots you don't take."

But 47 percent was still a shot. Heck, 24 percent was still a shot.

But this wasn't just a shot; it was an opportunity. I had the opportunity to live life without seizures again. I wouldn't allow the risks to cloud my optimism, not even for a second. In the past I had wondered what abilities I might lose if surgery went wrong. But my frame of mind now said, "What have I got to lose?" I had already lost my career and my ability to train hard for marathons —the two big things that motivated me to get up each day. But just as important as setting and meeting goals was the big thing I was missing out on—a personal life.

My mind flashed back to the last few weeks I had spent in Michigan.

If I said no to surgery . . .

No. No was not an option. I would live in fear every day that another seizure would strike. Eight hours of sleep 365 days a year wouldn't be a reality unless I wanted a new career testing mattresses. Not going to happen.

Epilepsy was an enemy that would lash out against me without enough rest. So who was I to doubt a team of epileptologists and neurosurgeons, with decades of combined experience? I was lucky to live close to two level 4 epilepsy centers in the Twin Cities, and the Mayo Clinic was just an hour and a half away. That's a huge advantage. A handful of states, including neighboring North Dakota and South Dakota, have none. Even more stark was the reality that most people with epilepsy live in low- and middle-income countries without access to good care, and up to 70 percent could live seizure free if properly diagnosed and treated, according to the World Health Organization.

My opportunity to possibly live seizure free was one that many people with epilepsy around the world don't have. In a sense, I had the mindset of both an athlete and a reporter—take opportunities when they're given to you. Dr. Penovich didn't need to do any convincing; I'm a realist and my logical brain prevailed.

Don't give up on yourself, Stacia.

I was lucky enough to qualify for a surgery with a high success rate. Settling for a life of more memory loss, of waking up each day with a good chance of forgetting what you laughed about with your sister or best friend the night before, wasn't an option.

Your life won't be forgotten by others, only you. Think about others.

Saying yes was only fair to my family and friends, who had been through a lot and deserved to stop worrying about me. Saying yes was my brain's way of asking for help. Surgery could hopefully end the daily fear of seizures and give me my freedom back.

Things wouldn't change unless I changed. Risks for further injury and future job discrimination would increase. Surgery could eliminate both.

I wanted my life back.

Doing is different than trying. You try skiing a black diamond or bungee jumping. You don't try brain surgery; you do it.

Sometimes experiencing something horrible can scare us enough to take a risk that might actually help. Breaking bones, suffering multiple black eyes, and face-planting into a brick wall didn't scare me enough. Getting lost while running didn't scare me enough. It took getting fired to truly absorb the fact that I couldn't outrun epilepsy.

The girl who had hidden and denied her seizures for five straight years—saying, "No, I'm fine; they aren't that bad"—now had a chance for a better life.

If I could wake up at 2:00 a.m. to run along dark streets not knowing when or where another seizure would strike, it seemed a little hypocritical to say surgery was too risky. It was only fitting that my answer should be a resounding "yes."

Two excellent neurosurgeons, Dr. Meysam Kebriaei and Dr. Mary Dunn, would perform my surgery.

The thought of saying "no thanks" seemed absurd.

My current memory problems made the decision easy. I wanted to stop frustrating friends and family during conversations. I wanted to stop filling scrapbooks with photos to remind myself of the fun I had while my eyes filled with tears because I was unable to remember.

Simply put, I wanted to reminisce again.

"Do you remember last year? That restaurant downtown we got drinks at, and the people across from our table?"

I longed for that kind of memory. One to laugh at with everyone else in the room, to laugh so hard my stomach would hurt. The kind that turns into high-pitched, almost unpleasant squealing because nobody can stop. My sister sometimes made me laugh that hard over simple, goofy things. But the topic of our laughter never stuck with me.

At that point in my life, I was smiling, trying to hide the frown inside, while everyone else was trying to catch their breath, nervous for me. I was surrounded by laughter that was contagious to everyone but me.

I wanted in on the memory. I wanted back into the moment.

Now, with surgery approved, the opportunity to protect my memories was up to me. The only way to do that was by placing my future in the hands of two skilled surgeons.

23

Back behind the Camera

Neuroscientists and doctors might call me naive for not truly understanding the potential effects of drilling my head open, mapping my brain, and removing a portion of it. But my naivety was to my advantage. I didn't want to know any more about a high-speed drill to my skull and a scalpel to my brain than necessary. Their confidence was reason enough for me to sign the consent form.

The people I met at the Minnesota Epilepsy Group and United Hospital gave me hope, and I chose hope over fear. Once I accepted that mindset, surgery became the easiest decision of my life, and making that decision helped clear the stress that was cluttering my mind. In its wake came a big idea, one that would draw on all my talents as a reporter and journalist: I would film a documentary about this experience.

The thought was so random it surprised me for a second, until I realized a documentary could educate the public. I tuned back into reality with Dr. Penovich long enough to say goodbye and left the hospital completely preoccupied with the possibility of a film. When we stepped outside, I called my family to quickly give them the news of the impending surgery, then turned back to my big idea. My mom recalls that I became interested in the documentary immediately after the appointment. "You didn't even want to take time to celebrate your surgery decision over lunch," she told me.

Within three hours, I sent off emails to Ken and my other journalism mentor, John Pompeo, a Detroit TV news videographer, asking for their thoughts on the idea. Their journalism experience was far beyond mine, and I trusted their judgment. My phone buzzed with matching responses. Ken's and John's offers to help would lead to the most meaningful job of my life. I was going to have brain surgery, and I would produce a documentary to share my journey. How's that for a big news day?

The last few hours started to sink in, and as I sat down to reflect, old memories surfaced. I had spent seven years telling other people's stories, and now seven months after being terminated, it was time to tell my own. Every interview—whether in an office, in a school, in a city building, at a home, or on a street corner—started the same way: get a close-up on the person's face, focus the lens, and press record. Now I'd put my own life into focus to show how a seizure could turn someone into a completely different person in mere seconds.

I've always been a somewhat private person and naturally reluctant to tell friends and coworkers about my seizures. But as a reporter, I understood how storytelling could educate people and help them understand nearly everything, if done well. If sharing the worst moments of my life with strangers across the world could spread awareness, that's what I would do.

But epilepsy has many faces and includes many people who understand what it feels like to be looked down upon. As I considered the social stigma surrounding epilepsy, my mind wound back to the football coach at my alma mater and the hateful comments he received from viewers and sports columnists.

"We've got a freak coaching the Minnesota Gophers."

"No one who buys a ticket to TCF Bank Stadium should be rewarded with the sight of a middle-aged man writhing on the ground."

Jerry Kill needed to be in the documentary. His decision to speak out about seizures took courage, and I was inspired by his example. He had partnered with the Epilepsy Foundation of Minnesota to increase epilepsy awareness education in Minnesota schools and help fund a wonderful camp for kids with epilepsy through the Chasing Dreams Coach Kill Epilepsy Fund. Through its executive director, I connected with Jerry and was thrilled when he agreed to be in the film.

This is actually going to happen!

Buying a new camera and gear was up next. I asked around for recommendations and bought one nearly identical to what I had used as a reporter. Ken connected me with a professional videographer to help shoot the interview with Coach Kill, and a few weeks later, I stepped foot on the University of Minnesota campus for the first time in years.

Nerves fluttered in my stomach as I opened the doors to the Bierman Field Athletic Building and approached the staircase. I had jogged up and down these steps hundreds of times on my way to practice. Now I paused briefly as I lifted my foot, wondering in that moment who else with epilepsy had climbed these steps? Jerry Kill and I couldn't be the only ones out of the thousands of athletes, coaches, and support staff over the years. If there were others, how many had tried to hide their seizures like we had? Would fellow athletes, coaches, and reporters have questioned their ability? Who, like me, would develop epilepsy later in life and assume that employers and colleagues would look down on them? And what had given me reason to think that way to begin with? Epilepsy is most common in children and older adults, but anyone can develop epilepsy at any age.

The videographer and I walked into Jerry's huge office, where memorabilia filled the shelves and desk. He greeted me with a big hug, instantly making me feel as though I'd known him for years. Once the camera started rolling, my questions flowed naturally. He gave me as much time as I needed.

We chatted and shared stories about our seizures and how people reacted to them.

"Why do you feel there is such a stigma around epilepsy?" I asked him.

"It's easier to say 'seizure,' 'seizure disorder,' than 'epileptic.' I don't know if it has to do with the brain, the mind, or it's the word," he said, gesturing with his hands. "And to me, a lot of it has to do with . . . the word, you know. Made you sound like a freak or something."

"Freak" was the word an anonymous person had called him in an email.

Then came the topic I really didn't want to bring up but had to.

The game two years ago against New Mexico State and the column that followed.

I didn't need to quote it. He remembered.

"How did it feel to hear a sports columnist say you should step down because of epilepsy? And not in a kind way?"

"Did it bother me? Yeah, yeah, I mean who wouldn't. I'm not that tough," Kill told me. "I'm not going to sit here and tell you I'm the super toughest guy in the world, I'm not. There isn't anybody that wouldn't bother. You know, I just didn't show it on the outside. Inside, it hurt. I mean why wouldn't it, you know, it hurts."

But he quickly followed up by saying he had met with the columnist and chose to forgive and forget. He also shared some sobering thoughts on how that one game began to change the conversation on epilepsy.

"I'm over it, done with it, move on. And those people, in a different way, helped epilepsy more than anything in the entire country," he told me.

I sat back in surprise and admiration for Kill. He recognized that negative publicity can sometimes lead to positive outcomes. In this case, it brought the brain disease we shared to the attention of thousands of football fans, even coaches.

"Two Big Ten coaches called me and said, 'Coach, you got to tell me, I don't know anything about epilepsy,' " he once said during a speech at an epilepsy event.

Kill became a national face of epilepsy. He spoke at events across the country, and he stood up for people who had stayed on the sidelines for so long, scared that friends, classmates, or coworkers would find out. People like me.

Coach Kill wanted to know my story, so I opened up to him about the last few months. His reaction was genuine.

"That was the best thing that ever happened in your life," he told me. "If that didn't happen you wouldn't be doing this. Someone's got a plan for you."

My chest instantly filled with emotion. The football coach at my alma mater had validated my mission, to help people understand epilepsy.

"Exactly," I replied with a smile.

We chatted some more as I glanced around his office at all the maroon and gold. The rich colors brought back a brief image of me donning the university colors at a home cross country meet. I smiled with pride as I pulled that snapshot out of my memory bank. Competing for the Gophers had molded me into the person who was now up for this new challenge.

Before epilepsy, my career had been my biggest focus. I dreamed of rising from one market to another, wherever life took me. I imagined I'd eventually settle down with a family, a house, and a dog. Epilepsy interrupted all those plans. But had I not moved past the humiliation and pain of losing my career, I wouldn't be able to start making a new plan. Coach Kill's comment was the pep talk I needed, an extra dose of encouragement to do the film. I would need it once again, a short time later, when it was time to turn the camera on myself.

When the documentary began to materialize, so did the realization that I would need to show one of my seizures in it. The thought terrified me, but if I was truly going to be an advocate for increasing epilepsy awareness, educating people could only happen if I was vulnerable. I requested video of a handful of seizures from my recent EEG monitoring at United Hospital. At that point the closest I had come to watching one was in Dr. Smith's office, but glimpsing just a few seconds had traumatized me, so he stopped the tape. My idea had been to show just one of the seizures in the film. But my mentors Ken and John said that wasn't enough.

"The viewer needs to see you watching your seizure for the first time, meaning you need to be on camera in front of your computer," Ken said. John told me the same thing.

I froze.

Taking their advice was something I'd always been happy to do. Combined, they've got a few more decades of journalism experience than I do. But the way people had described my seizures, the screaming and waving, had me convinced that watching myself have one on camera was a terrible idea. Not knowing exactly what would unfold, I decided to suck it up and get out my camera. I was back in Minneapolis, living with my college teammate Christine, and I picked a sunny afternoon when she wasn't home to set up the camera and computer. Normally, I'd have someone else control the camera, but with a hint of what lay ahead, the idea made me extremely self-conscious. I had to do this on my own.

With the lens pointed at the side of my face and the camera rolling, I clicked on the folder containing one of my seizures. An image of a stationary bike filled the computer screen. My body tensed, but I told myself to calm down since I was on camera.

"Just based on what people have told me, that I scream and stuff, I'm kind of nervous, but I think it's good for me to know," I told the camera.

After a big breath, I pressed play.

You'll be fine.

The whirling sound of the stationary bike filled a hospital room outfitted with video EEG monitoring. Just minutes earlier, a nurse had walked me down to the bike.

"OK, this is number one."

With electrodes dangling from my scalp and the EEG tech fixing a bad wire, I started to pedal apprehensively. The conditions were just right for a brainstorm—sleep deprivation, reduced medication, and exercise.

Would it be jamais vu? Déjà vu? Flickering lights? Or no aura at all?

I watched my own face intently.

The hospital room's camera captured what unfolded next. My legs aren't in motion for long before my eyes glaze over and a wave of confusion crosses over my face.

I start rubbing my arm, and just when the EEG tech gently moves the wire over my shoulder, the seizure suddenly spreads. It hijacks my motor function, and I thrash my arms up and down and yell, all while continuing to pedal as usual. Staring at the computer screen, watching myself have a seizure for the first time, my surprise turns to shock, then to tears, as I try to grasp the sight. Here I am, caught up in a brainstorm, with no conscious idea that I'm throwing what looks like a temper tantrum.

"My mom comes in and she has to see that," I said through my tears, pointing to the monitor. "She's talking and saying my name."

My poor mom—the seizure she heard in the Michigan hospital hallway and now had to witness for twenty-eight intense, excruciating seconds. The yelling soon subsided, and my arm movements slowed to a stop a few seconds later as I caught my breath and looked around, trying to make sense of my surroundings. The entire seizure lasted about thirty-five seconds, and my feet never stopped pedaling. The seizure had overrun my vocal cords and arm motion but not my legs and feet; the disconnect in my brain amazed and frightened me.

My hands shook as I reached over to turn off the camera, and then I tucked them under my chin and closed my eyes. Mortified. I was mortified. My thoughts swirled. The video played over again in my mind as I sat there. How could I be pedaling normally while waving my arms in large circles and screaming, all at the same time, without realizing it?

Everything was completely out of sync. It would have been hard enough doing that while conscious. The brain truly is a computer. I wondered if I waved my arms in circles in the same way when seizures had struck while I was out running. I didn't really want to know. A few more clips were in the file that my clinic had sent over.

The emotional part of me said, "No! Do not put yourself through watching another one." But the curious side of me reasoned, "Relax, you've already made it through one. How much worse can it be? Surely, they don't all look exactly like that."

Before I could change my mind, I double-clicked on another video. This time, I was talking on the hospital room phone when the neurons started misfiring. Fear suddenly filled my face as I looked down at the pen in my hand. "What's this?" I shrieked, as if I was holding a snake. My eyes widened, and my arms started swinging for a good thirty seconds before the seizure died down.

"OK, that's enough. I've seen enough," I said in disbelief as I closed the file.

These are worse than I thought they'd be. Why do most of my bizarre seizures look similar each time?

I learned that seizures often have a stereotypical pattern, so both their duration and features are predictable. Later I interviewed Dr. Penovich to help me understand why my behavior was consistent with epileptic seizures. She said epileptic seizures start and end on their own, with a recovery period, and they are unprovoked. "That's very different from somebody who is having those behaviors due to other reasons, such as taking substances, drugs, or having a psychiatric issue."

Leading up to surgery, I busied myself with documentary work, but one date stayed on my mind. The Michigan Emmy Awards were being held on June 13, 2015. For the first time in my reporting career, I had entered a compilation of stories and was surprised to be nominated in the "Video Journalist" category. The category honors reporters and photojournalists who shoot all or most of their own video and write and edit their stories. The ceremony in Detroit was streaming live, so I sat down to watch that night on my computer.

When my category came up, I took in a few shallow breaths as the announcer read off the nominees. When they called my name as the winner, I laughed with shock into my computer. My face flushed, and my smile didn't leave it until John—my mentor in Michigan— walked onstage to accept the Emmy and speak on my behalf. He had volunteered to receive the statue if I won, but he never mentioned what he would say. I sucked in my breath in nervous anticipation as the ballroom went quiet and he started talking.

"She was forced out of her job because of a disease. And in less than forty-eight hours she's going to be having surgery to fight this beast. And I'd like you for a moment to imagine the job you love to do is taken away from you because of something you have no control over."

Tears of gratitude spilled out, forcing me to turn up the volume to drown out my heavy breathing. John spoke with a calm sense of authority, his tone very direct.

"You might be a little miffed, a little hurt, think like, 'I can still do this.' So, I know she's watching, and I know this means a lot because it validates that she should still be doing this. And hopefully she can battle this disease and conquer it and get back to doing what she is so good at. Thank you on her behalf, and I know this is going to make her day and hopefully help her recovery."

Speechless and emotional, I sat there as the room erupted in applause, trying to absorb the powerful words he spoke to the hundreds of TV journalists, photographers, and producers in attendance.

"It validates that she should still be doing this."

I glanced down at the editing sequence on the tool bar.

"Yes it does," I said with a wide smile.

My goal was to get the documentary aired on PBS. I did the math.

Lengthwise, it would be equivalent to roughly thirty-six news stories. A fifty-four-minute documentary was a huge challenge, and that's why I was already enjoying it. The structure would come once all the interviews and transcribing were complete. So far, Jerry Kill, me, members of our families, and Kate, as well as our doctors, were helping educate people and bringing awareness to epilepsy.

One person would be both on camera and behind the scenes—my sister, Sara. We interviewed each other, and she used her amazing design talents to create some of the graphics for the film.

With the outline in place and some interviews complete, it was time for me to take one of the biggest opportunities of my life. I had qualified for this first surgery to map my brain. Now the upcoming iEEG would confirm where the seizures were starting and how close they were to my critical functions. The results would either move me along to the second surgery or end my best shot at seizure freedom.

24

Brain Mapping

"You were very calm the evening before in the hotel room as if nothing were to happen," my dad recalled.

My parents and I were getting ready for bed at our downtown Saint Paul hotel, a few blocks from United Hospital. The 4:30 a.m. alarm would be the earliest one I'd set since my 2:00 a.m. wake-up calls as a morning reporter in Michigan. I was teaching my parents a few basics on my video camera. The plan was for them to capture me walking into the hospital the next morning for the documentary. Shooting video was second nature to me, but it was brand-new to them. The white balance, zoom, and focus buttons all got a few run-throughs. It was fun to share some of my profession with them, a nice distraction from what would soon unfold.

The surgery was out of my control; dwelling on it felt like a waste of time. Instead, I drifted off to sleep thinking about the camera angles I would need in the morning. The alarm woke me instantly. I got up and changed into comfy clothes—shorts and a zip-up. Breakfast, coffee, and water weren't allowed before surgery, so I grabbed my backpack and camera and ushered my parents out the door. After giving them a brief rundown outside the hotel, I handed my mom the camera, clipped the microphone to my shirt, and did a mic check; then we strolled down the quiet sidewalk along Seventh Street. At five-thirty, the sun began making its way up and over downtown. The walk was peaceful. As we approached the hospital, my mom lifted the camera, hit record, and asked how I was feeling.

"OK, here we go. The hospital entrance is right here. I'm ready to go, I'm ready to go," I said, my voice filled with happy energy.

The camera didn't lie—the smile on my face was genuine. I was just so relieved this day had finally come.

Once indoors, we headed to the surgery center, checked in, and took a seat in the waiting area. I thought that moment would be a great time to ask my mom how she was feeling. My upbeat attitude hadn't waned, and I figured she would be happy too. The waiting area was empty, so I turned the camera back on and zoomed in on her face to focus the lens. A view that close gave me a window into her light blue eyes and made me pause. For the first time I could actually see the anxiety in her gaze. For the last eleven months, my physical and mental health was all my mom could focus on. And it took a camera lens for me to see how much that stress took a toll. Downplaying the seriousness of my seizures had blinded me to how worried my family had become. No matter how I was feeling, my answer was the same:

"Mom, I'm fine, stop worrying."

"Yes, I'm sleeping better, don't worry," I had tried to reassure her.

After I lost my job, I repeated similar things to my parents multiple times. "Don't fly out to Michigan. I'll be fine here for another month until my lease ends."

Red puffy eyes and thinning hair are easy to hide over the phone, but did I ever have a meaningful face-to-face conversation with my mom or dad about the seizures? Did I actually look into their eyes? No. I hated talking about epilepsy, so I made eye contact only occasionally, told them the truth like I promised, but then moved on to a new subject as soon as possible.

I didn't want to see the concern on their faces. It would hurt too much. But eye contact holds people accountable, and at that moment, my mom was holding me accountable. Her eyes revealed to me what a child's serious medical condition can do to a parent. I didn't have the option to turn away, so I took a big breath and held out the microphone with a big smile.

"OK, mom, it's the morning of surgery. How are you feeling?" I tried my best not to sound like a reporter.

A soft but tense smile appeared.

"Nervous," she said in a timid tone I hadn't heard before, meeting my gaze. "It's pretty hard. It's hard," she said quietly, nodding her head and looking down.

Tears filled her eyes, and she looked back up, tried to smile, and then looked away.

I had never seen her cry.

"It's going to be fine. I'm really glad this is happening. I'm glad that you had all the tests that you had so we can do this today, but . . . ," she paused, taking a breath before meeting my gaze again, "it's hard."

Her response caught me off guard. I had expected her to be excited like me, but I was too distracted with the surgery to sit there and really digest her feelings. I hugged her tightly, doing my best to convince her that everything would go great. It was my turn to be the reassuring caretaker for a moment.

It didn't cross my mind in that moment to interview my dad next, and I wish I had. He's easygoing and kind and never worried openly around me. His calm helped offset my mom's nervousness, but I never thought to ask about his feelings. The time and place of that interview with my mom was a stark reminder that a successful surgery was not all about me. I wouldn't be the only one to get back their quality of life. And success was the only outcome I could envision when the nurse called us into the preoperative room.

Thoughts of a failed surgery never occurred to me; with the documentary in the works, my mind was swimming with creative ideas. Many people have asked me since then if the idea of brain surgery made me nervous. The starting line of races made me nervous, as did live shots in my early reporting days. That's because I was mostly in control of what happened in those situations. The documentary was a gift that took my mind away from the what-ifs. And, thankfully, I wouldn't be the one holding the scalpel.

Dr. Kebriaei greeted my parents and me to review the risks, then stated he couldn't promise a successful operation. He would perform a craniotomy to place electrode strips and a grid—about the size of a Post-it note—directly onto the surface of my right frontal and temporal lobes.

The invasive brain surgery was not without risks, which included hemorrhage, infection, bleeding, swelling, and stroke.

My mom turned to me in disbelief. "If you are feeling anxious or apprehensive, you certainly aren't showing it." She still managed to give her written and verbal consent along with my dad, and I quickly gave my consent, wishing I could have been hooked up to the anesthesia on the spot. The moment came soon enough. After a lengthy surgery prep, the clock struck 7:30 a.m. Time for surgery number one.

The plan was to map my frontal and temporal lobes with a grid and electrode strips so that Dr. Penovich and her colleagues could identify the seizure onset zone and the EZ. In addition, functional cortical stimulation would map my brain functions. Their review of the brain mapping reports would determine if the epileptogenic zone could be safely removed without damaging important brain tissue. If so, I would proceed with surgery number two, the resection. Once I was intubated, sedated by anesthesia, and lying on my back on the surgery table, Dr. Kebriaei and Dr. Dunn started the craniotomy.

First, they placed the back of my head into a head frame, turned my head to the left, placed a shoulder roll underneath my right shoulder, and shaved off a long strip of hair. Then they brought out a laser pointer to register images into a neuronavigation system called BrainLab. My doctors had already uploaded my three-dimensional MRI images from earlier that year, so a laser scan of my face captured my cranial structure and aligned it to the 3D MRI model of my brain. BrainLab also had a virtual map of the operating room; once the surgery table was aligned with the map, the software could track the surgical instruments and my brain throughout the procedure in real time.

Once my skin was sterilized, Dr. Kebriaei followed the path the razor had shaved off with a blade, cutting a large, reverse question mark on the right side of my head. The incision only went deep enough to pull back my scalp, and he started at my hairline, smack-dab in the middle of my forehead, right where I often parted my hair. Dr. Kebriaei guided the blade backward about seven inches, before turning right and following a path straight down to my ear, stopping right above my ear lobe. That was the reverse question mark. Next, he pulled my skin back toward my right eye to reveal my skull.

He then identified the area where he wanted to perform the craniotomy, which would be about five centimeters in diameter. First, he drilled small holes, called burr holes, into my skull. He used a very thin saw, called a craniotome, to cut straight lines from hole to hole until the bone flap could be lifted and set aside until the operation was complete. A craniotomy is a highly delicate operation because of the chance of cutting too deep and damaging the brain surface. Under the bone sits the dura, the strong, fibrous protective covering of the brain, which the surgeons carefully opened. Then came the next challenge—placing electrodes onto precise areas of my brain's surface.

The Post-it note sized grid was placed directly over my temporal lobe, and three electrode strips were fitted in surrounding areas of my right temporal and frontal lobes. The surgeons then connected yellow wires to the grid and electrodes and tunneled them up toward the scalp incision at the top of my head, where they protruded from the skull and would later connect to a small device that would map my brain. Dr. Penovich tested the electrodes to make sure everything worked before Dr. Kebriaei closed the dura, replaced the bone flap with titanium plates and screws, and stapled the skin back. The center of my head reminded me of a train track when I saw it later.

It was midafternoon by the time nurses wheeled me to the post-anesthesia care unit, then to the neurological intensive care unit. I arrived in my own room later that evening, where I would stay for the next twelve days. My mom was anxious to see me, but there were so many postoperative tasks to complete that the nurse gave her only a couple of minutes. Because of the grid, a nurse would always be with me, 24/7. Falling during a seizure fresh off brain surgery could be fatal.

My room was equipped for epilepsy monitoring with a video camera on the wall, which, paired with the iEEG, would capture any seizures that occurred post-surgery. My brain seemed to wait

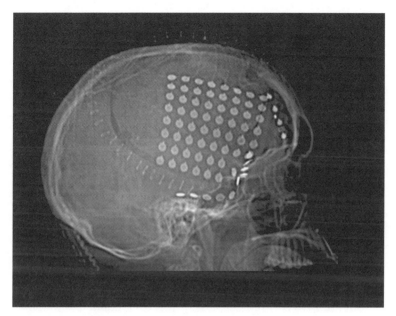

An image captured from a CT scan shows the subdural grid that was surgically placed onto my brain to map my seizures.

only long enough for me to get situated before neurons started misfiring. I have no recollection of any of these seizures, but my medical chart included detailed notes.

The first seizure started just before 7:00 p.m., when I was lying flat on my back with my eyes closed for an EKG to check my heart's electrical signals. I started grasping at my clothes and smacking my lips. This focal impaired awareness seizure was taking over part of my right temporal lobe and continuing to spread across other portions of the grid.

Fifteen seconds later I loudly and randomly asked, "Is this a girl?"

I appeared confused by what was going on with my heart. Things calmed down, but not for long.

About thirty minutes later, I was still on my back with my eyes closed. Fentanyl and hydromorphone were running through my veins to try to tame the massive pain already developing from the craniotomy. I was extremely groggy, but the headaches I remember quite well. Meanwhile, my seizure medication had been reduced.

The iEEG suddenly lit up—spiking was coming from the right temporal lobe again, but this time it was spreading farther across the grid and over to my right frontal lobe. The seizure continued to build until it finally jolted me out of my drugged-up state, and I started screaming and waving my arms for ten long seconds.

Things worsened.

An hour later, according to my medical notes, the nurses were talking with me, and I was feeling nauseous from all the medication. My third and final seizure of the night started off by spiking again in my temporal lobe, and I become less talkative, though I did respond to a question. The spiking increased and fear filled my face.

"What?! No!" I yelled, then screamed loudly. Apparently, I tried to bite the nurse caring for me. Talk about bizarre.

But after twenty-four seconds, it was over, done, just like that. I snapped back to baseline immediately and could speak clearly, identify objects, and respond to questions. A craniotomy and some intense seizures. That's a lot for a brain to handle in one day. I'm guessing I slept a long time following that final seizure.

My brain was too foggy to remember much of anything, but I do recall how friendly and supportive the nurses were; having a calm, consistent voice by my side following a seizure was reassuring. I'm less sure they felt calm around me the entire time.

Thinking about it later, visualizing my body flipping on a dime and my mind suddenly overcome with fear to the point of screaming, it seems unreal. How can I share the same body with a complete stranger who acts nothing like me? A person might say, "Stacia, that wasn't you. It was just your brain sending mixed messages." But those were still my arms and legs and my voice acting out for twenty-four seconds.

It turned out that the iEEG monitoring of those three awful episodes captured some crucial and unexpected details that the previous EEG tests could not see. The instigator was not my frontal lobe after all. Seizures were forming and firing in my right temporal lobe for about twenty to thirty seconds before recruiting enough nearby neurons to spread to my frontal lobe. This is the brain's control center, and once the mixed messages started flying, my motor functions went haywire.

The muscle artifact shown in previous tests truly was hiding crucial information.

Would future seizures show the same pattern? It took twenty-one hours to get an answer, which proved to be no. The following seizures over the course of five days were polar opposite.

First, I had one of my typical auras, which lasted just seven seconds.

The next day, a seizure recorded on the iEEG didn't change any of my behavior. Nurses were walking and talking with me while neurons short-circuited for thirty-eight seconds. I didn't miss a beat. My speech, walking, and behavior were all normal. This would happen again. I was having seizures without even noticing.

In another episode, I was resting in a chair while a brainstorm lit up my temporal lobe for forty-nine seconds, with no clinical signs of the seizure until right at the end when I opened my eyes and looked up. As I read through my medical notes, the stark realization hit me. How often had I been having seizures in Oregon and Michigan without any clue? My heart was skipping beats, and my brain was misfiring neurons, and I was running around with a video camera at work, oblivious to it all. Now that's bizarre.

In the final recorded seizure from the iEEG, I was sitting in the same chair and talking normally, but I quickly became less responsive and started smacking my lips. Twenty seconds later I asked, "Who won?" A nurse asked me to repeat the color "purple," and I did, very loudly. Once the seizure ended, I was back to normal right away.

Sitting here today, reading the iEEG report, I wish I could get inside my brain in those moments. What compelled me to say randomly, "Who won?" Why did I repeat "purple" so loudly? To my relief, everything about my behavior was consistent with epilepsy—the repetitive movements (smacking my lips and grasping my clothes), the hyperkinetic movements (kicking my feet and thrashing my arms), the unusual speech, and the sudden sense of fear.

These seizures were all starting in the right temporal lobe and spreading to the right frontal lobe.

Eight days into my hospital stay, it was time for mapping my brain functions—functional cortical stimulation. An EEG technician sent brief electrical currents to dozens of contacts on the grid and electrodes to map precisely where my language, motor, and sensory functions were stored. This allowed my doctors to observe how areas near the seizure onset reacted. If a current caused my speech to become jumbled, then that area was deemed important for language. If any parts of my body started or stopped moving with the current, then that area was responsible for movement. If any of this happened, it could limit how much of the seizure focus surgeons could safely remove, or it could end a potential resection altogether.

In the end, brain mapping was a success. After ten long days, my doctors had the content they needed. All the seizures that were recorded formed in my right mesial temporal lobe, then rapidly spread to my frontal lobe. That was the moment the overactive neurons put my motor functions into overdrive.

I stayed put in my hospital bed while Dr. Penovich presented my results to her colleagues at a meeting. They changed course. My right mesial temporal lobe was officially the generator, not the frontal lobe, and no critical brain function was standing in the way; as a result, my surgeons would perform the standard in temporal lobe epilepsy—a cortico-amygdalohippocampectomy to remove the front portion of the temporal lobe and the entire mesial structure, which includes the hippocampus and amygdala.

The frontal lobe—which helps control thinking, organizing, movement, and problem-solving—could stay intact because it wasn't within the epileptogenic zone. I was too drugged up to recall my reaction to finding out the second surgery would occur, but my parents remember my instant excitement. They said I had no hesitation.

Candidates for a resection have seizures developing in one area, like the right temporal lobe. Dr. Smith told me the brain has reserve—in my case, the left temporal lobe—which is why I was a good candidate. "That small portion where the seizures are coming from can be removed, with very minimal change in overall function, and you've got, in a sense, a cure."

Dr. Dunn explained the resection surgery to me when I interviewed her for the documentary. "If we take it [the EZ] out, we take out the generator. So with the generator missing, the seizures stop."

The generator allowed the seizures to spread to the frontal lobe and cause the kinds of physical behaviors we were seeing. But though it may sound simple on paper, the EZ isn't a perfectly outlined area for surgeons to tackle. Leaving just a tiny bit of tissue intact could keep the seizures coming.

I didn't focus on what might be left behind, only what lay ahead.

The resection was scheduled for the following morning. Once I was back on the operating table and Dr. Kebriaei registered me to BrainLab again, he reopened my bone flap to access the grid and electrodes. Those came out first, and then he brought in the microscope and resected four centimeters of the inner part of my temporal lobe. Then, under microscopic magnification, neuronavigation guided him to also resect the entire amygdala and hippocampus.

My hippocampus, my amygdala, and part of the temporal lobe were packed in formalin and sent to a pathologist, who scanned them and ruled out masses and cortical dysplasia, an abnormality where the top layer of the brain does not form properly. To my surprise, the pathologist didn't find any evidence of scarring in my hippocampus. How could my memory be terrible if my hippocampus looks fine? My new epileptologist, Dr. Jessica Winslow, explained one possibility.

"We always keep in mind that only a sampling of the tissue that was removed will be looked at under the microscope," she told me.

Dr. Bertram said that if my hippocampus truly wasn't impacted, and surgery stopped the seizures, then some bad actors were generating the seizures that were not visible on imaging but had been removed during surgery. That's why the resection covers more than just a tiny area that seizures fire from. Surgeons performed a cortico-amygdalohippocampectomy for a greater chance of seizure freedom. Leaving the hippocampus intact would leave the potential for neurons to start misfiring months or years out.

Waking up to the beautiful June sunrise the next morning after surgery felt strange. Twelve days had passed since I arrived at the hospital, and now I was a completely different person in one sense. Some of my brain was gone. Painkillers were on full throttle, but underneath the discomfort and fogginess was a nervous curiosity.

Am I supposed to feel different?

I don't feel any different.

A few important pieces of my brain are missing. How can I feel like the exact same person? Maybe this is my postoperative state and I'll start feeling different once the morphine wears off.

I scanned the room and immediately recognized my parents.

Whew, good start!

The following day I was still in a daze.

Sara, Mike, and Tom soon arrived, but my mom said I was too drugged up to hold a conversation.

But talking with young, healthy people gave me hope that I'd soon be able to remember conversations just as they could. Here I was, thirty years old, recovering from two brain surgeries, and thus far doing great. Time would tell if the surgery was 100 percent effective, but I just felt so lucky to have made it this far. My voice choked up with emotion when Sara took out the video camera and asked how I was feeling.

"This is probably the worst pain I've ever been through in my life, but I just have to count my blessings, because many people don't get to do this, but the goal is for me to be seizure free, and I think we're on our way to that happening."

Sara returned the following day with a gift that made me both laugh and cry. A section of my hair had to be shaved off for surgery, so now I needed a way to hide the bald spot.

"I brought you some hats. I think this one would be good for fall." My sister is the stylish one and has a hat for every season.

"Thank you, my wonderful sister, for taking care of my head," I said with a smile.

She kissed my gauze, then my nose, and said goodbye. Finally, the time came for the big reveal. Nurses unwound the thick headwrap to unveil staples and the result of twelve days of glue and multiple hands touching my head, without a drop of shampoo or water. My matted hair was so greasy that pulling the strands apart was impossible.

My fingers grazed the fresh row of staples that lined the incision. The small clumps of hair that had fallen onto my Michigan apartment floor eleven months earlier due to stress had left a few small bald spots. Comparing bald then to bald now made me laugh out loud. There wasn't enough hair to cover this size of bald. Only a hat could do it, and now I had a few.

After twelve days in the hospital, my doctor cleared me for a little stroll down the hall, and this was a big deal because crossing the room by myself wasn't allowed while the grid was in. Cautiously I got out of bed, stretched out, and took some steps around the room.

My brother Tom returned, and we took slow steps down the hospital hallways with a nurse. Moving my entire body again, though slowly, felt amazing. My gait, movement, and awareness were all intact, which was a relief. All the tight muscles and tendons were free to loosen up, but I definitely noticed they had atrophied a little after two weeks in bed. Five pounds had vanished from my body, all muscle. Ugh. But I brushed it off.

Muscle will be easy to gain back.

That turned out to be very wishful thinking. But, thankfully, I was still me.

The final visitor on my last day in the hospital carried with him something that brought a huge smile to my face. Tony Pompeo is my mentor John Pompeo's cousin and someone I'd never met before. He lives in the Twin Cities but was in Michigan recently to see family, and John sent him home with a gift. He introduced himself to my family and then held up a bag with a big grin and took out a gold box, about the size of a large shoebox, and handed it to me.

The smile didn't leave my face because I knew what was inside: my first Emmy Award, which John had accepted two weeks earlier.

The gleaming gold statute was heavier than I expected, and its weight made it that much more significant to me. Seeing my name engraved on an Emmy was surreal. Then came a flashback to watching the awards ceremony and John's speech: "She was forced out of her job because of a disease. And in less than forty-eight hours she's going to be having surgery to fight this beast." The smile left my face briefly. But then perspective set in. As strong as the physical pain was at that moment, it didn't cause tears. But the emotional pain I felt eleven months earlier could have filled a bucket.

Look where you are, Stacia. The termination letter brought you right here, to this hospital bed, and surgeons just removed brain tissue and altered your life forever. What would your life be like today, at this very second, if you hadn't moved back to Minnesota?

Tony and I chatted for almost an hour, and then we took a picture so I wouldn't forget his face. My spirits and health had improved enough to leave the hospital. Dr. Kebriaei and my nurses gathered by my bed for a picture, which I now treasure, then released me with a prescription for painkillers, aftercare instructions, and a reminder card to get the staples removed from my head. That was one reminder I wouldn't need.

Dr. Penovich decided to continue my seizure medications, because there still was no guarantee the surgery had been successful. She told me seizures are not uncommon for a year following surgery, as my brain healed. Part of the healing process was to avoid anything that would put pressure on the brain, and I left with a list of tight restrictions for the next six months: No bending down (my dad would tie my shoes for me). No driving or heavy lifting—heavy was anything over five pounds, including a gallon of milk. I had no complaints; the thought of lifting anything at that moment made my head hurt.

But no running or strenuous exercise was a tough pill to swallow. After six months, I could start easing back into training very slowly, but nothing at my usual intensity for a full year. Six months

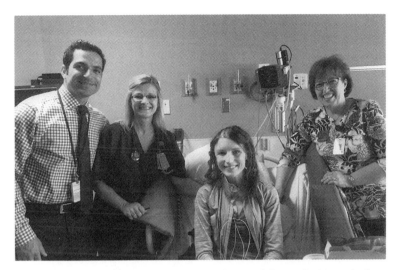

My surgeon, Dr. Kebriaei, and the nurses who cared for me during and after surgery.

with no exercise bummed me out, to say the least. *Shut up. Again, perspective.* I had gone through four months of testing to qualify for a surgery that many people don't get a chance at. *Don't complain or take any chances of upsetting your brain. End of story.*

After the final hugs and goodbyes at the hospital, my parents helped me to the car. They would take care of me for the next six months. We pulled into my childhood home on Maple Avenue after the six-hour drive. When I stepped through the side door, relief washed over me. The kitchen to my left and the cozy family room to my right brought me back to high school. I loved this house. At eighteen years old, I had skipped out the same door and driven the same six hours south to Minneapolis, excited to start college. I left home young and optimistic, with no lived experience yet that would prove the old adage "Life isn't fair." Now, twelve years later, I wasn't allowed to drive for at least three months, and my upstairs bedroom would be my haven to sleep for eight to twelve hours every night to curb headaches as my brain healed.

Looking in the mirror each morning brought a small laugh and sense of awe. Thick staples lined the incision from my forehead

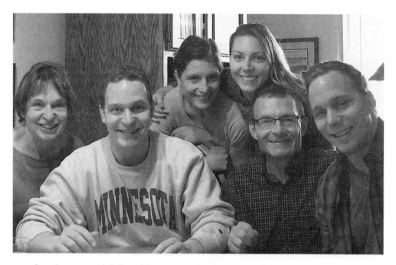

My family at my childhood home in Thief River Falls, Minnesota, after my surgery.

down and around my ear, and for the first few weeks, the right side of my head was swollen to the size of half a small orange. A room across the hall became my office, with a big wooden desk overlooking the tree-lined street. Concentrating on anything, including the documentary, was impossible at first because the headaches were so intense. Even with 20/20 vision, life was blurry, and the computer screen strained my eyes. I forced myself to ease back into life slowly.

My path to normal was dictated by excruciating pain, and only frequent rest and short walks around my neighborhood at dusk lessened the constant pounding in my head. But that was enough for me. Summers in Minnesota were beautiful, and I looked forward to even a short stroll and the opportunity to call friends. The walks were a break not solely for my eyes but also for my entire body. Every time I breathed in the fresh air, it reminded me how lucky I was to be able to stroll down the street.

But there was no guarantee that I was seizure free yet. Getting enough sleep was easy at that time, but knowing a seizure was always lurking kept me on guard every day.

25

Caregivers' Worry Never Ends

The strange taste came on slowly, making its way up from the back of my throat. My back went rigid as I sucked in my breath and sat up straighter at my desk. About three months out from surgery, I was feeling pretty good. The headaches had all but disappeared, and each passing day made me more hopeful that the surgery had cured my epilepsy.

At this moment, though, my entire body was on high alert, trying to identify this bitter flavor and how it had invaded my mouth. I hadn't eaten anything recently, and I didn't feel strange anywhere else. My mind quickly scrolled through the other aura symptoms I'd learned about.

Taste . . . taste . . . ick.

Yuck.

Yes, that's it! Some people with epilepsy get a metallic taste aura.

I had never actually tasted pennies before, and I wasn't about to try now, but it felt like a decent comparison. What else could it be? I stood up, half believing, half not believing it was a seizure. The awful taste disappeared, and my neurons behaved well for the rest of the night.

Let it go. It could have been anything. If it happens again, take it seriously.

A few months later the strange taste returned. I froze, now accepting the fact that it could be a seizure. I told myself to breathe, hoping that it would go away again. By instinct, I glanced up at the kitchen light with trepidation, its brightness illuminating the entire room. Then I looked down and slowly back up again, narrowing my eyes.

"Don't you dare, do not flicker," I whispered.

I observed my arms and hands, the desk. Everything looked

familiar. So did the furniture at my parents' place. I looked up at the light again and took a long, shaky breath as the metallic taste dissolved under my tongue.

Thirty very long seconds had passed, without me falling apart.

Still, there was a good chance that was a seizure. I informed Dr. Penovich, and she upped my medication slightly. Those were two of a handful of metallic taste auras I had the year following surgery. They scared me to my core; I never knew where they would lead or whether I would lose consciousness. I still experience this aura occasionally today. But the taste comes and goes, and I remind myself each time that surgery had removed that part of my brain.

Quit overthinking it.

Though those initial auras were disappointing, overall my surgery was a huge success. I could live with a gross taste for thirty seconds once in a while.

I decided to title the documentary *Brainstorm* and continued plugging away at writing, shooting, and editing throughout the summer. The participation of my medical team was essential, and, happily, Dr. Penovich, Dr. Dunn, and Dr. Smith agreed to interviews.

Three months after surgery, my dad drove me the 880 miles to Grand Rapids. At his office, Dr. Smith greeted me with his familiar warm handshake. He had shown me a few seconds of one of my seizures when I lived in Michigan, but I had quickly asked him to stop; it scared me. Now that I knew what a few looked like, I wanted him to describe a seizure with the EEG waves to show what was happening inside my brain in real time. Seconds later he pulled up my chart on the computer and picked out a seizure to watch. He chose a seizure that he had called a "somewhat unusual event" in my medical records. As it turned out, "unusual" was an understatement. Without knowing what exactly was on the video, I asked my dad for help with setting up the camera, and Dr. Smith walked over to a huge monitor.

"OK, go ahead," I said, and my dad hit the record button.

The seizure Dr. Smith selected starts with me eating lunch on a hospital bed. Within seconds, the seizure begins creeping in. The nervous look on my face signals the first visible clue something is off. I softly swear, then take a bite of food.

"You take the food out of your mouth because you know something's not right," Dr. Smith explained, pointing to my face on the video.

Just then, the seizure spreads and takes all control of my body. I'm no longer consciously aware of what I'm doing. My face looks exasperated as I start tapping my fork hard against the hospital tray.

"You didn't have any reason to start tapping your fork. This is just one of those repetitive mannerisms that can happen as the brain is starting to short-circuit," Dr. Smith explained, pointing to my brain waves spiking on the EEG monitor.

On the video, I exhale heavily and hit the fork harder and faster before ending with three angry taps. Then comes the worst sound I've ever heard—a loud, piercing scream.

As I watch my body—the one I am sitting in at this moment, the one I've lived in for thirty years—suddenly succumb to a storm of misfiring neurons, I'm mortified. It's like a scene out of a horror movie, with an unknown actress taking my place in that hospital bed. My arms wave back and forth, and I scream again, then again. Though it looks like I'm awake as I yell, wave my hands, and kick my feet, I have no idea that I'm doing what I'm doing. And then after one minute, it's over, like a wailing baby who finally runs out of steam. The actress vanishes, and I slowly look around the hospital room, depleted and confused.

A nurse approaches my bed and gently asks, "Do you know where you are?"

Dr. Smith observes my blank facial expression in the video and then turns to me to explain.

"For a while, you're not going to necessarily be able to respond and answer questions, because it's almost like a rechargeable battery that is discharged and needs to be recharged," he said.

The nurse asks again: "Can you tell me where you are?"

Twelve seconds later, my brain works hard to put enough pieces of the puzzle together to quietly respond, "Hospital."

Soon after, I can follow her other commands.

I was grateful to Dr. Smith for his time and left Michigan feeling much more confident about the documentary. Explanations about my seizures from my doctors not only provided vital educational content for the film but also helped me understand how my seizures could look so bizarre, as Dr. Smith had described them. The long drive back to Minnesota gave me time to sort through all my footage. Jerry Kill and me, our families, two epileptologists, and one surgeon. But something in the story was missing.

A child.

Both Jerry and I were adults. But nearly half a million children suffer from seizures in America, and I was curious about how families tackled epilepsy.

But who could I interview?

I gave my brain a minute to scan its reserves. This would be a good test of what memories I held onto after surgery. Then it hit me. Two years ago, I came across a story about a ten-year-old boy named Billy Drash from Atlanta. Coach Kill had invited Billy and his father, Wayne, to practice the night before the 2014 Epilepsy Awareness game versus Ohio State. In a heartwarming video, Wayne captured his excited son entering the practice facility and getting a warm welcome from Coach Kill.

"How you doing?" Kill asked, extending his hand.

Billy slapped it with a wide smile.

Kill laughed. "You doing all right?"

Then he handed him a Gophers helmet.

"See what it says? 'You're my idol. Coach Kill.' "

"Is that for me?" Billy asked.

"Yes, yes it is," responded Kill with a chuckle.

Billy grabbed the helmet and pulled it over his head.

"There you go. You look pretty good in that," said Kill.

I laughed as I watched the sweet young boy interact with Coach Kill. Their connection was instant. I got in touch with the Drash family, who agreed to an interview, so I grabbed my camera gear and hopped on a flight to Atlanta in late October 2015. Wayne and Billy gave me a warm welcome, along with Billy's mom, Genny, and his sister, Emma. Billy has a learning disability on top of his epilepsy, so Wayne and Genny shared the highs and lows of his day-to-day life. It was eye-opening and humbling to see a child go through the stress of seizures, to know that his parents make trips out of state to find the best doctors. I didn't even know what a seizure was at Billy's age.

Then I put myself in their shoes. Epilepsy would have completely altered my family's life if my seizures had started at a younger age. The closest epileptologist to Thief River Falls was nearly six hours away, as was a level 4 epilepsy center. Suddenly, my struggles didn't seem so big. I couldn't help but reflect on all that my parents had been through over the last five years. Every caregiver's role may be very different, I realized, but they're very similar in the end. Wayne and Genny worried about Billy at school, and my parents worried about me biking and walking to work. An unpredictable disease like epilepsy, one that can turn deadly under countless circumstances, often leaves loved ones on edge.

As my mom wrote to my coworker Kate, "I go into the station's website daily to see if she made it to work."

In the throes of epilepsy, my family's daily stresses were the furthest thing from my mind, as was the danger I faced. Until I lost my job, I was invincible.

////

I came to a stop, a little out of breath but thankful to be moving again. Dr. Penovich had restricted running for a full year following surgery, and now it was the summer of 2016, and I was granted the freedom to pick up the pace again. For someone who had run down a basketball court, across a tennis court, and around a track her entire life, this thirty-second jog brought back a flood of memories in an instant.

The film's creative process was helping me heal faster, I believed. Writing and editing video, with plenty of small rest breaks, forced me to think creatively both on paper and about the editing timeline. Ken reviewed script edit after script edit, and I printed out multiple pages with his new suggestions. Finally, it was time for voiceover. Ken connected me with a recording studio, and two years after voicing my last TV story, I stepped up to a microphone. The words came out, but my pitch was too high. After a few more attempts, I finally got into a rhythm. Once finished, I was on my way to a final rough edit. I loved the new challenge brought by the writing and editing journey. Epilepsy had become a topic I cared deeply about, and the project gave me a purpose to get up each day and work late into the night.

The end result was more than I could have hoped for. Twin Cities PBS acquired the broadcast rights to *Brainstorm,* and their executive director of programming set an early November 2016 deadline for me to submit the final edit. That date happened to be right before the New York City Marathon, a race that I couldn't run but my sister could. Her mission in participating was far more important than a time on a stopwatch. Sara was competing for me on a team called "Athletes vs. Epilepsy," a devoted group of four-teen runners from across the country who together had raised over $50,000 for the Epilepsy Foundation. I was committed to being there to cheer her on in Central Park.

After Sara put her final touches on the film in postproduction, she took off for New York City. I then worked into the wee hours, watching the entire film twice to catch any last errors, before sub-mitting it to Twin Cities PBS and caught a flight the next morning. Once I landed and hailed a cab, the driver sped through the traffic, weaving between lanes against a chorus of car horns. My stomach lurched with every sharp spin of his wheel, like I was on a ship in rough waters. By the time he pulled up to the Airbnb on a quiet street on the Lower East Side, I was close to vomiting.

But my nausea soon disappeared once I hugged my family. We visited for a bit before heading to the marathon expo.

Sara and I jogged to the "Athletes vs. Epilepsy" prerace pasta dinner to meet the other athletes and their families. The team din-ner was at the classic Italian restaurant Carmine's. My longest run since surgery had been just six minutes, but my feet fell in line with Sara's and felt strong for the one-mile jog from the expo to the restaurant. At the family-style dinner, we traded stories with the other athletes while sharing some of the best food I've ever eaten.

My goal was to jog to a spot where I could catch sight of Sara and cheer her on. The next morning I bundled up, stepped out into the crisp November air, and took the subway to the Queensboro Bridge. Sara would be on her sixteenth mile by then, and I thought she could use some encouragement. I tracked Sara's race, and when she ran by, her tank top was hard to miss. The white mesh was emblazoned with the words "Athletes vs. Epilepsy." My heart swelled with pride as she raced by.

While most marathons have sections along the route where the crowd thins out, the New York City Marathon is packed nearly every step of the way, with each borough bringing their own unique music and enthusiasm to cheer on the runners. My body was so energized that I didn't even realize I was jogging while cheering. I made my way to meet my parents in Central Park, where the final three miles of the race took the runners through a long finish line filled with lots of excitement, fun signs, and loud cheers. Sara finished within her goal time and set a personal record. My parents and I navigated through the crowds and light rain to meet her. She was hard to find among the other runners, all wrapped in giant blue parkas.

"You're amazing, Sara!" I cried, hugging her. "Thank you for racing for me!"

I had never imagined I'd be happily cheering someone else from the sidelines. Though I so wished to have run with her, I was content that day. A much bigger wish had come true—I jogged around all morning without a single seizure on limited sleep. Surgery had worked.

26

Brainstorm

Brainstorm premiered on Twin Cities PBS on November 20, 2016. The Epilepsy Foundation of Minnesota sponsored a screening of the film that same week, followed by a Q and A. Almost immediately following the premiere, and in the months after as the film continued to be aired, viewers emailed me with their own stories. I could relate to so much of what they had to say. They talked of hiding their epilepsy from friends, of stresses related to their jobs, of feeling embarrassed by their seizures, and of the pain of witnessing a loved one's seizures.

"I stumbled on your movie at 3 a.m.," one viewer wrote, "when I was unable to sleep due to stress from the possibility of losing my job. Within five minutes of watching, I was in tears. FINALLY I found a movie that puts EVERYTHING I have tried to explain to so many people throughout my life into a platform I can share. Every feeling you described, I shared with you. Every tear that you shed, I shed with you."

Up to that point, I had only met a handful of people with epilepsy, so these messages left me humbled. *Brainstorm* went on to air on public television stations across the country, and I was, quite simply, floored by the response. One viewer wrote to me about having to retire from a fulfilling career in the military, of putting off surgery on his left temporal lobe. Seeing the documentary made him reconsider. The irony of someone brave enough to fight in combat but too afraid to share his epilepsy with anyone but his family was not lost on me.

A common thread running through many of the letters was fear: both of when a seizure might strike and what epilepsy can do to relationships. One viewer in her early sixties told me about several sisters and family members who are afraid of her because of her seizures. Another worried for his nine-year-old son following a traumatic brain injury. But the film also brought hope to many living with epilepsy. "For the first time, I realized that what I have is NOT weird or freaky, and there might be help for me," a viewer wrote.

We all yearn to be understood. Releasing *Brainstorm* into the world brought me closer to understanding the reality of epilepsy in people's lives. Soon enough, I would get the opportunity to hear their stories face-to-face. Before making the documentary, I never could have predicted that I would use a microphone for anything other than broadcasting the news. That all changed when I recorded the voiceover narration for *Brainstorm*. Nor could I have predicted what would come after the documentary. Invitations arrived from cities across the country, not to report or to broadcast but to simply talk. From the heart.

The first time I really felt the magnitude and true relevance of epilepsy in America was a few months after I finished the documentary. UCB, a global biopharmaceutical company that produces a number of antiseizure medications, invited me to Los Angeles to share the patient's perspective at their annual Patient Impact Meeting. The company wanted to show their sales team how patients live daily, some controlled with medication, some not. This was my first big speaking engagement, and I was nervous.

We gathered in a ballroom the size of a small theater at the JW Marriott hotel. Before I spoke, Dakar De La Cruz, UCB's senior brand manager for epilepsy patient initiatives, took the stage to introduce me. Three huge monitors surrounded the stage behind her as she pressed her mini remote and stepped aside. The numbers "1 in 26" filled the screen. I knew those numbers well. One in twenty-six people will develop epilepsy at some point in their lives. The statistic astonished me when I first heard it in 2015. Before then, I never bothered to look at the stats because I wanted nothing to do with epilepsy. Seeing "1 in 26" is like seeing many other medical statistics. They're shocking. Heart disease, diabetes, opioid overdoses—we let these things sink in for about a minute and think of all the people they affect. But the shock value starts to wane when we see the same statistics repeatedly. Without a personal story attached, the growing number of people in pain is difficult to grasp.

But "1 in 26" will never lose its shock value for me. Dakar's presence was powerful, and so was her message. I don't remember her speech word for word, but the comforting words of Maya Angelou convey its lasting power: "People will forget what you said, people will forget what you did, but people will never forget how you made them feel." Dakar reminded her team that "1 in 26" is a profound number to patients like us. For that one person, epilepsy is life-changing. Medications too can change lives. On the screens she displayed photos of people with epilepsy who chose to share their stories in UCB's *Epilepsy Advocate* magazine. People just like me.

I was sitting off to the left in the front row, looking up as she pointed to a person on the large screen. The person was both a stranger and someone familiar whom I could identify with immediately. I am one of the "1 in 26." Just like him, just like the other people she showed. Merely a year and a half earlier I wasn't the only one who took meds and still had seizures, not the only one living an unpredictable life. I had an intractable case of epilepsy that medication could never control. And for that reason, I would head to a surgery table for a resection.

I saw their faces. They were different than mine, yes, but our eyes connected. Eyes can tell you so much about a person. They lit up bright for the camera, but I knew that behind the lens, those eyes had seen a lot of darkness. For some, the darkness would arrive abruptly, with a seizure taking over multiple parts of their brain, knocking them to the ground in convulsions. For others, the clouds moved in first, with an aura that stopped them in their tracks and filled them with fear, warnings that their bodies would soon succumb to the electrical storm firing in their brain. By looking at the screens, I couldn't know what kind of darkness those eyes had experienced, how often it struck, or how damaging the seizures were. Nor could I know if epilepsy had caused other darkness that could creep in, like depression.

Looking up at those people on the monitor changed my perception in seconds. I never thought of myself as a statistic. Dakar was onstage saying no one with epilepsy should think that way. We were more than a number, she went on to say, and her sales team needed to know that people were relying on ASMs every day to live. With that, she introduced me as one of the nearly three million American adults living with epilepsy.

I took a few deep breaths.

Pull yourself together. You need to speak eloquently.

I stood up and stepped onto the stage, feeling confident and realizing at that moment how important my message really was. One in twenty-six people translates to one in twenty-six families, including my family, the Kills, and the Drashes. With epilepsy, we all lived in an unpredictable and frustrating world. We were all very different, yes, but also the same. Sharing clips from *Brainstorm* with the strangers in front of me felt odd at first. These were people who knew nearly nothing about me until that moment. But I had nothing to lose; I could only win if they learned something that day.

I don't remember at what point Dakar's earlier words hit me onstage. This time, though, I couldn't hold the tears back. I really tried, but when it comes to health issues and the people impacted by them, I lose my composure. This was a huge stage, the lights were bright, people had come to hear about my journey, and all I could think of were the people in that magazine, struggling with epilepsy. My emotions tumbled out.

"I'm sorry, I didn't plan to cry," I told the crowd.

I never do, but I wear my heart on my sleeve, and that day my heart was breaking for the fifty million people worldwide who don't get a chance to be heard. They don't get to explain why medication is vitally important to every second of their day, why seizures are scary, and why the recovery from one is sometimes worse.

Seeing their faces on a huge screen hit me. I turned back to the microphone.

"Those advocates are heroes," I told the crowd.

They were my heroes because I knew their pain and because they also realized it was time to share their stories with the world. I wiped away my tears to continue talking, knowing I had the responsibility to share my story with the medical and epilepsy communities, employers, anyone willing to learn about epilepsy, or anyone faced with adversity.

I'm fully aware that there are many children and adults whose epilepsy cannot be controlled, despite their attempts at surgery, implantable devices, numerous medications, and other methods. I've met them and it's heartbreaking, but I'm hopeful that neuroscientists will continue to develop new therapies so that one day everyone's epilepsy can be treated successfully. In the meantime, I hope people will seek out the best care available and be confident in trying a new treatment.

In 2015, I was one of the lucky people who qualified for brain surgery and was even luckier to have had a successful outcome.

My mom reflected on my experience best: "Sharing this journey is your payback for doctors giving you your life back." I'll never take my brain surgery's success for granted. Never. Every week I cut my ASMs to the exact dose needed to fill my pillbox to keep that awful metallic taste at bay. Washing down those pills twice a day washes away the doubts. Those blue oval pills are my confidence markers for the day.

Epilepsy has left behind a few visible reminders that it once controlled my life. The bathroom mirror creates random moments to reflect on my good fortune. Raising my hand to brush my hair offers a glimpse of the long scar along my forearm. It turned white long ago, a reminder that external scars heal over time but leave their mark as a warning. Our bodies are strong, but they are not invincible. They need to be protected. On my head, my hairbrush sweeps over the thick, question mark–shaped indent carved into my skin. Every morning, I part my hair to cover the scar, which is too large to ever disappear. But that's fine with me.

Washing my face gives me a glimpse of what that incision took and left behind. My right temple has a slight indentation from the resection, and I can feel the titanium plate and screws that repaired my skull. One of the screws peeks through the skin. A permanent bruise there reminds me that my head took a beating.

I glance over to my left lobe, where the scar over my eyebrow remains from my second seizure in college when I fell off my bunk bed and cut my eye on a desk.

On the left, a reminder of what used to be, the scar marking the beginning of a rough journey to get to the right side. And on the right, a reminder that every rough journey eventually comes to an end.

My eye catches one last scar, under my left collarbone. The large incision made to insert the pacemaker is the reason I made it this far. It's a reminder of a silver lining. Mine is in the form of a thin silver oval, a battery keeping my heart up to speed. The testing in Michigan is undoubtedly the reason my heart is beating today. Sometimes a trip to the hospital is a gift in disguise.

With epilepsy, as with many obstacles, you learn how to deal with the unexpected. Seizures hit whenever they feel like it. You'll fall down—really hard—but you'll learn how to get back on your feet. And to keep getting back up. You'll learn to stay up, go to school, and go to work. You'll gain the confidence to run, hike, and live your best possible life. But it won't be easy. Epilepsy will take you on a different ride every time.

////

I turned the corner onto my parents' property and looked at my watch. My sister and I had just finished a four-mile walk. I thought back to the mornings when I didn't feel it was worth it to lace up my running shoes for less than four miles. Never again will I brush off a four-mile run. But never again will I put running ahead of health. A healthy body is a gift. A healthy mind is an even greater one.

There's no doubt that the determination and resilience I developed in athletics got me through my job loss and surgery. One phrase you'll hear repeatedly from coaches and athletes is "Don't give up." But it's more than that.

Don't give up on *yourself*.

Resources and Further Reading

According to the Epilepsy Foundation, one in twenty-six people will develop epilepsy at some point in their life. Approximately 3.4 million Americans have epilepsy, and for about one million of them, medication does not control their seizures. More people live with epilepsy than with Parkinson's disease, multiple sclerosis, and cerebral palsy combined. The following organizations provide more information about epilepsy, publish some of the leading medical research, advocate for patients and their families, and work hard to end the stigma of epilepsy.

American Academy of Neurology
https://www.aan.com

American Epilepsy Society
https://www.aesnet.org/

CURE Epilepsy
https://cureepilepsy.org/

EpilepsyDisease.com
https://epilepsydisease.com/

Epilepsy Foundation
https://www.epilepsy.com/

Epilepsy Foundation of Minnesota
https://www.epilepsyfoundationmn.org

International League Against Epilepsy
https://www.ilae.org/patient-care

Jeanne A. Carpenter Epilepsy Legal Defense Fund
https://www.epilepsy.com/legal-help

For employers, educators, and readers who are interested in streaming options for the epilepsy documentary *Brainstorm* or who would like to purchase a DVD copy and access an accompanying discussion guide, please visit https://brainstormdocumentary.com.

Understanding epilepsy—or the brain, for that matter—isn't easy, and research continues to grow each year. Still, there is much that isn't known, which can make it a challenge for patients and caregivers just starting out after a diagnosis. According to the World Health Organization, the cause of the disease is still unknown in about 50 percent of cases worldwide. Readers interested in learning more about epilepsy can find valuable information in the following books.

Epilepsy: A Patient and Family Guide. 3rd edition. By Orrin Devinsky, MD. Demos Health, 2008.

Epilepsy, 199 Answers: A Doctor Responds to His Patients' Questions. 3rd edition. By Andrew N. Wilner, MD, FACP, FAAN. Demos Health, 2008.

Epilepsy Explained: A Book for People Who Want to Know More. By Markus Reuber, MD, et al. Oxford University Press, 2009.

Epilepsy in Children: What Every Parent Needs to Know. By Orrin Devinsky, MD. Demos Health, 2015.

Living Well with Epilepsy and Other Seizure Disorders. By Carl W. Bazil, MD, PhD. HarperResource, 2004.

Navigating Life with Epilepsy. By David C. Spencer, MD, FAAN. American Academy of Neurology and Oxford University Press, 2017.

Seizures and Epilepsy in Children: A Comprehensive Guide. 4th edition. By Eileen P. G. Vining, MD, et al. Johns Hopkins University Press, 2022.

Other memoirs about epilepsy include *Chasing Dreams: Living My Life One Yard at a Time,* by Jerry Kill (Triumph Books, 2016); *A Mind Unraveled: A Story of Disease, Love, and Triumph,* by Kurt Eichenwald (Ballantine Books, 2018); *The Sacred Disease: My Life with Epilepsy,* by Kristin Seaborg, MD (independently published,

2016); *She Danced with Lightning: My Daughter's Struggle with Epilepsy and Her Boundless Will to Live,* by Marc Palmieri (Post Hill Press, 2022); and *A Smell of Burning: A Memoir of Epilepsy,* by Colin Grant (Vintage, 2017).

For this book, I relied on the expertise of my doctors and specialists I've met over the years. I also consulted the following published research.

The Mayo Clinic offers a concise summary of frontal lobe seizures, including symptoms and causes, diagnosis, and treatment: https://www.mayoclinic.org/diseases-conditions/frontal-lobe -seizures/symptoms-causes/syc-20353958. See also "Recommendation for a Definition of Acute Symptomatic Seizure," *Epilepsia* (April 2010), https://doi.org/10.1111/j.1528-1167.2009.02285.x.

For a discussion of memory loss and epilepsy, see "Remote Memory in Epilepsy: Assessment, Impairment, and Implications Regarding Hippocampal Function," *Frontiers in Neurology* 13 (April 2022), https://doi.org/10.3389/fneur.2022.855332; and "Remote Episodic Memory Deficits in Patients with Unilateral Temporal Lobe Epilepsy and Excisions," *Journal of Neuroscience* 20, no. 15 (August 2000), https://www.jneurosci.org/content /jneuro/20/15/5853.full.pdf.

Research on the postictal state (the state of altered consciousness immediately following a seizure) is published in "After the Wave Subsides: Post-ictal Effects," *Epigraph* 22, no. 2 (Spring 2020), https://www.ilae.org/journals/epigraph/epigraph-vol-22 -issue-2-spring-2020/after-the-wave-subsides-post-ictal-effects; "Aggression and Violence in Patients with Epilepsy," *Epilepsy Behavior* (May 2000), https://www.epilepsybehavior.com/article /S1525-5050(00)90061-1/pdf; "The Postictal State—What Do We Know?" *Epilepsia* (May 2020), https://onlinelibrary.wiley.com /doi/10.1111/epi.16519; and "Biting Behavior, Aggression, and Seizures," *Epilepsia* (May 2020), https://onlinelibrary.wiley.com /doi/10.1111/j.1528-1167.2005.58404.x.

Information on mood disorders and behaviors observed during frontal lobe seizures, as well as a helpful glossary of terms used to describe seizure signs and symptoms, can be found in "Emotion and Mood Disorders Associated with Epilepsy," *Handbook of Clinical Neurology* 183 (2021), https://doi.org/10.1016/B978-0-12-822290-4.00008-6; "Directed Aggressive Behavior in Frontal Lobe Epilepsy: A Video-EEG and Ictal Spect Case Study," *Neurology* (November 2009), https://doi.org/10.1212/WNL.0b013e3181c2933f; and "Seizure Semiology: ILAE Glossary of Terms and Their Significance," *Epileptic Disorders* (June 2022), https://onlinelibrary.wiley.com/doi/pdf/10.1684/epd.2022.1430.

Research on epilepsy surgery, including studies from the Mayo Clinic and the Cleveland Clinic, is available in "Epilepsy Surgery Outcomes in Temporal Lobe Epilepsy with a Normal MRI," *Epilepsia* (August 2009), https://doi.org/10.1111/j.1528-1167.2009.02079.x; "Seizure Outcome and Its Predictors after Temporal Lobe Epilepsy Surgery in Patients with Normal MRI," *Epilepsia* (July 2011), https://onlinelibrary.wiley.com/doi/10.1111/j.1528-1167.2011.03091.x; and "Surgical Outcomes in Lesional and Non-Lesional Epilepsy: A Systematic Review and Meta-Analysis," *Epilepsy Research* (May 2010), https://doi.org/10.1016/j.eplepsyres.2010.02.007.

Acknowledgments

Most of the pages in this book wouldn't exist without the help of my family, friends, and coworkers, who filled in all the memory gaps that epilepsy stole from me.

First, to the person who pushed me to write this book. I was reluctant to share the details of my bizarre seizures and the end of my reporting career, but after two years my sister finally convinced me that doing so could help the public understand the many faces of epilepsy. I'm beyond thankful to Sara for believing in me from the beginning and for providing invaluable input to my first draft. She's the best sister I could ask for, and I'm beyond appreciative of her support.

To Dr. Edward Bertram, Dr. Arthur Cukiert, and my current epileptologist, Dr. Jessica Winslow, with deep thanks for answering my long list of medical questions, particularly on memory, mood, and behavior during seizures. Their knowledge made this memoir an educational resource, and I appreciate their time and contributions very much.

To Jacquelin Cangro, whose editorial feedback early on helped me develop the big picture and establish the vision for the book. Thank you for the guidance.

To Diane Stockwell, for the second edit and for finding areas for improvement.

To my editor at the University of Minnesota Press, Kristian Tvedten, whose edits sharpened every chapter of the book and made these pages immeasurably stronger. Thank you for asking so many questions about epilepsy to add more depth to the book.

To Anne Taylor, for the valuable suggestions and the meticulous copy edit. Thank you for all of your attention to detail.

To my publisher, the University of Minnesota Press, for seeing the importance of educating readers about epilepsy and believing in me as a first-time author. I'm honored to be published by my alma mater.

To the Epilepsy Foundation's Jeanne A. Carpenter Epilepsy Legal Defense Fund. The foundation's prompt work in connecting me with attorney Joey Niskar right after my job loss was important for my mental health at that time. Joey's dedication to my case and willingness to work pro bono still amaze me. Securing my work file helped me piece together the two-hour chaos that took place in my brain that day and not only brought me closure but made this memoir possible. I will be forever grateful for the Epilepsy Foundation's help.

To Kate, my friend and coworker who recognized the seriousness of epilepsy early on and didn't settle for my excuses. Kate's emails to my mom jump-started the path to better treatment, and her early ideas for improving this manuscript were spot-on. I'm so lucky to know Kate as a friend and journalist.

To Kara and Christine, my longtime friends, for sharing details about my health that I had no idea about all these years later. They both helped me connect the dots between my early seizures, memory, and mood. I'm grateful for their friendships then and now.

To my friends and coworkers in Michigan—Sarah, Alana, and Chad. I couldn't have asked for better people in my life when my seizures became known. Thank you for not treating me any differently and for the laughter, the car rides, the acts of advocating for me at work, and the generous emotional support, especially in the days following my termination.

To my journalism mentors, Ken Stone and John Pompeo. Without *Brainstorm,* writing a memoir never would have crossed my mind. The documentary laid the framework for the book; I wouldn't have watched my seizures or learned details of my epilepsy without the film. Thank you for believing in the importance of sharing my story from the start.

To the five doctors who treated my epilepsy, whose combined

expertise stopped my seizures and gave me my life back: Dr. James Kiley, Dr. Brien Smith, Dr. Patricia Penovich, and my surgeons, Dr. Meysam Kebriaei and Dr. Mary Dunn. I am forever grateful. Their dedication to improving patients' lives is no doubt the reason I'm alive today.

And, finally, to my family—Mom, Dad, Sara, Tom, and Mike. I didn't understand the amount of worry I put on everyone until I started this memoir. There aren't enough words to express how lucky and thankful I am to have had the level of support they showed me then and continue to show me now. I owe everything to my family.

Stacia Kalinoski is an Emmy Award–winning TV news journalist. When a seizure ended her career in 2014, she chronicled her journey with epilepsy and brain surgery in the documentary *Brainstorm*, which was broadcast on PBS stations and nominated for a regional Emmy Award. She now shares her story of resiliency as a motivational speaker.